Vienna's Waiting

Georgia Huston Weston

First Edition

Copyright © 2011 by Georgia Huston

All rights reserved, including the right to use or reproduce this book or portions thereof in any form whatsoever without written permission from the publisher except in the case of brief quotations embodied in critical articles or reviews.

Teen Pain Press
21545 Yucatan Avenue
Woodland Hills CA 91304
www.cosworthpublishing.com

ISBN: 978-1-970022-11-7

For information regarding permission, please send an e-mail to *office@cosworthpublishing.com*.

I dedicate this book to anyone who is in pain.
You are not alone.

Preface

It may seem self-centered for a seventeen-year-old girl to write a book that's all about herself. I know there are those who have suffered more – but this is my story. I'm writing it – digging as deep as I can and reliving my darkest experiences – because I feel with all my heart that this will help someone.

I'm not the only kid who's gone through this, and I know first-hand that the worst thing of all was feeling alone and lost.

If my story can help just one other kid, then I will be happy. If kids in pain can relate to what I went through, I will be satisfied. I need to let those kids know that they are not crazy.

They are not alone.

Chapter One

"Name and age, please?"

"Umm..." I close my eyes and grimace, turning my face up toward the ceiling. The fluorescent lights are glaring down on me. I can feel their dirty looks. I clench my fists so tightly my fingernails make marks in my palms as I tap the counter in rhythm.

"Miss?" The lady behind the desk, whose name tag identifies her as Sue, still doesn't even look up from her computer. *Can she not hear the helplessness in my voice; the chattering of my teeth?*

"Yeah, sorry umm... Georgia Huston. I'm fourteen." I turn around to look out the glass door. *Where is my dad?*

"Okay, G-e-o-r-g-i-a H-o-u-s-t-o-n, age fourteen...."

"No, it's Huston, H-u-s-t-o-n." If I had a dollar for every time someone made that mistake I could buy this hospital and run it the way I wanted to. I could get every doctor here to care about me and to heal me from this mysterious illness.

"Oh, I'm sorry, Miss Huston. Please have a seat and we will be with you as soon as possible."

As soon as possible – those words mean absolutely nothing to me anymore. Before all of this happened, I probably could look past the vacant stare and the monotone voice; look past it to a promise that they meant. Now, I know the truth. The fact is, in half an hour there is going to be a shift change, seven p.m. exactly. When the shift change happens, Sue will log off her computer, push her chair in, grab her coat and purse, walk out, and never think about me again. She will walk off and live her life while I sit here in the waiting room, waiting. It's not that Sue does it on purpose, or in spite. It's just the way things are.

Sue #2 plops herself into the receptionist seat, logs into her computer without even looking around the waiting room at the agonized faces, all yearning for medical attention.

I want to lie down, but there are armrests separating the long couch into individual seats. I would usually not want to press my face onto the plastic seat where ill strangers' butts have been, but at this point I don't care.

The world is spinning so fast that even though I'm sitting, I feel like I'm about to fall over. My heart is beating so fast I honestly think I am going to die, which of course makes it beat even faster. I feel blood rushing into my head and I cannot focus on one thought at a time; it feels like a million incomplete thoughts are all coming in at once and it is the most frustrating feeling in the world. My hands and feet are cramping at the same time, to the point where I cannot move them.

I look down at the paperwork on the clipboard.

a) I cannot make out all the little symbols that make each word; everything is too blurry.
b) Even if I could make out a word, the words combined wouldn't make any sense in my tornado mind right now.
c) I can't even hold onto a pencil, much less write legibly.

I toss the clipboard onto the seat next to me. Even though I cannot read the questions on the standard medical forms, I know exactly what they are asking. Besides my name, address, and insurance information, I know that on the second to last page there is an outline of a body where I am supposed to mark where my pain is.

There is an outline of a person standing, looking straight ahead. I'm supposed to mark on the body where my pain is, but that image is not of someone going through pain. If the outlined person was feeling the way I am, its head would be dropped so low you couldn't even see its neck. It wouldn't be standing upright, it would be sitting, legs bent wide apart, head in hands, and shaking. Yes, it would be shaking uncontrollably; shaking out of pain, out of helplessness, and out of fear.

I know on the bottom of the last page there is a scale with faces ranging from smiling to crying, and that I'm supposed to mark where my pain lies. Hmmm... look at my face and you can tell me. *Where does my pain lie?* Is there a face on the scale that has sweat pouring down its cheeks, its jaw clenched as it grinds its teeth, and its eyes closed because having them open is just as scary as the endless darkness that it sees when it closes them? I don't see a face on the scale that illustrates where my pain lies. Sorry.

My dad rushes in from parking the car, scanning the waiting room.

He finds me cowering in the corner. "Did you sign in?"

I nod, closing my eyes, crying. He hands me my three pacifiers throughout this whole experience; my Burt's Bees Chapstick, my stress ball, and my iPhone with the pink case.

I put my headphones in my ears and blast "Vienna" by Billy Joel. It's an old song that not many kids my age know, but I know that song by heart. I listen to that song on repeat for hours at a time. That song made me fall in love with music and got me attached to songs. I don't know what it is about that song. Maybe it's his cool, old fashioned voice or his smooth, effortless lyrics that mesh together so easily it melts my heart. To this day, hearing that song always makes me cry. Each line seems to signify something different about how I'm feeling. I can usually get lost in the song, but now I can't.

Now all I can think about is how I am going to die. I'm going to die right here, in the waiting room at the UCLA hospital. My story will be in the newspaper tomorrow: TEENAGE GIRL DIES DUE TO UNKNOWN ILLNESS.

How will people feel about my death? Guilty; they will probably feel guilty. They should feel guilty, ignoring me out here like they always do.

I open my eyes just long enough to see the floor of the waiting room. When I close my eyes, the green checkered patterns are still engraved in my mind. I open them again to see my anxious dad pacing back and forth in the back of the room. That is by far the worst part about this, waiting.

Every tick of the clock and every janitor cart that rolls by sinks me farther and farther into my panic attack. I can't even recognize the song I'm listening to anymore, my body is beating to its own rhythm. I look over at the nurses with long fake nails, talking and chewing their gum. *Is that really more important than helping us out?* My body and mind build with frustration and anxiety. *Why isn't anyone helping me?* I hear a siren in the background. *Take me with you.*

Blood rushes to my head; everything goes black.

I wake up in a wheelchair, but still in the waiting room. *Really?* I passed out in front of a bunch of doctors and they still don't take me in? They simply rolled me in the corner, but don't worry, they will be with me as soon as possible.

Another hour goes by, Billy Joel being my only companion. I don't care what anyone says, he is speaking directly to me.

Slow down, you crazy child,
You're so ambitious for a juvenile
But then if you're so smart
Tell me why are you still so afraid?....

Slow down, you crazy child. How can I slow down when my mind is racing so fast I can't even keep up with it? It doesn't matter how ambitious I am, I'm still stuck in an ER waiting room. If I'm so smart then why can't I control my own body? That, Billy, is why I am so afraid.

"Georgia Huston?"

My head shoots up as my dad rushes to help me up. He is always one step ahead of me. We follow the voice to a small room with the door cracked. The light is so bright it takes a while to get used to, especially with my splitting headache.

"Please have a seat," the little man in the scrubs says while he motions to the foldout chair, not looking up from his computer; *big surprise*. He asks me for my age and some other basic questions. He sticks a thermometer in my mouth and starts to slide the blood pressure cuff over my left arm, but stops. "Excuse me, Miss. Can you please take off your sweatshirt?" *Are you kidding me? It's like ten degrees in here.* But, without saying a word I pull it off, trying not to mess up my hair too much.

My panic attack is gone, leaving me beyond drained and tired. It feels like I am in one of those horror movies where your body can't move but you can see, hear, and feel everything. That means I can see the reflection of the computer screen in the glasses of the man in the scrubs. I can hear the clicking of keys as he types my information into the hospital network. I can feel my arm hair being pulled as he pinches the wristband onto my arm.

"Okay, thank you, Miss Huston. If you'll have a seat in the waiting room, we will be with you as soon as possible."

Of course you will.

I want to go home so badly. The panic attack is over; *so why am I still here?* My dad forces me to stay to see a doctor. He wants answers. He wants his daughter's bizarre pain explained to him. He deserves that much; *doesn't he?*

I put my face up against the cold window, Billy in my ear, and I drift off to sleep.

"Paulina Jackson."
"Hannah Graver."
"Adam Faper."
Another hour goes by. Maybe two.
"Leah Boomer."
"Georgia Huston."

I hear it, but I don't wake up all the way. My sleeping hours have been on such an odd schedule I can't really control how I end my dreams anymore to wake up.

The next thing I know, I'm being wheeled into another bright room – no, a bright hallway. My vision is blurry; my eyes are so puffy and watery. *Wait, does this mean I'm going to be seeing a doctor?*

Now I'm being lifted by a very strong nurse, and gently laid down onto a bed. I open my eyes as my dad places my three pacifiers next to me on the white sheets. This can't be right, this isn't a room; this is just a hallway. Tons of people are rushing by me; I don't feel very comfortable here. I'm in everyone's way – a scared girl on a random bed in a busy hallway.

Every time I hear squeaky footsteps pressing into the hard, cold hallway floor, I look up. I look up to see mothers crying, sick children sleeping, and fathers pacing.

I go back in and out of sleep, losing track of time. I wake up just long enough to get hopeful as a doctor walks in my direction, and just long enough to be tormented as he walks past.

After what seems like forever, a doctor finally comes for me; only me.

"Hello, I'm Dr. Thirteen. Where is the pain?" he says, obviously only half interested. He is looking down at his clipboard.

"My back and leg," I say helplessly. Maybe he will be the one; the one to know what's going on. *Dr. Thirteen, be my hero.*

"Which leg?" he asks, scribbling on his clipboard.

"Right," I answer. Thinking about it makes it hurt worse.

"What part of your back?" Another scribble.

"Lower back, always lower."

"Any previous injuries that could have caused this?"

"No."

"On a scale of one to ten, one being no pain and ten being the worst, where is your pain?"

"Twelve."

"Okay, tell me if this hurts."

Dr. Thirteen has me lie down and starts to feel my right leg, watching my face for any signs of discomfort. I don't show much. When he goes to my back, again I don't feel as much pain as I should be with a finger probing my most sensitive spots. That's the thing, the pain is not really determined by the pressure I put on my leg or someone poking my back; it's more on the inside.

"Okay, Miss Huston, I'm going to order some X-rays and then we will have a look." *Yeah, good luck with that.*

"No need," my dad says politely as he places an intimidating stack of big manila envelopes on the hospital bed.

"What's this?" *Oh, Dr. Thirteen... meet Jimmy Huston; a.k.a. Mr. Prepared.*

"Her MRIs, bone scans – latest X-ray was taken last week so I don't think there's a need for another today." *You tell him, dad!*

Dr. Thirteen takes a few of the X-rays out of the envelope and examines them. "I want to take some from a different angle."

"What are you expecting to find?" my dad asks, not rudely, just trying to get information.

"I'm not sure. That's why we're going to take a look."

Oh, naïve Dr. Thirteen. You're right; this X-ray machine is a very special one, way different from all the others. The others are out to get me, hiding the problem on purpose. This one, this one will find it.

I get wheeled up to the X-ray room. "Any chance you might be pregnant?"

No.

They have me get into a paper-thin "gown" that I have to hold shut. I walk to the cold, dark room in just my socks. The X-ray technician is cute – this is really embarrassing. I regret not putting on makeup.

It doesn't hurt to get X-rays, everyone knows that, but what hurts are the positions they put you in for the X-rays. The room is so cold I'm shivering, but I know I need to stay still.

"Okay. If you go back to your bed we'll get these processed and to Dr. Thirteen as soon as possible," the cute technician says. He probably doesn't think I'm cute at all. *Who would?*

How do I get back to my bed? I turned left, right? I don't remember passing this painting or this security desk. This nurses station seems familiar, but they all look the same. Everything here looks the same.

I'm lost.

I can't ask anyone where I belong because there's no room number they can direct me to. *Can you help me find the bed in the hallway with the white walls and nurses?* They would look at me like I was crazy.

But I am crazy, remember? I'm feeling pain that no doctor can find, not even the best ones in the state. Unless my pain is more advanced than any research or machine in today's state-of-the-art medicine, I must be crazy.

After what seems like an eternity of wandering around long hallways into dead ends and DO NOT ENTER signs, I find my dad.

A little later, Dr. Thirteen comes back with matching manila envelopes. My dad and I make hopeful eye contact.

"Well," Dr. Thirteen starts, "we took X-rays of both your mid to lower back and your right thigh. I'm afraid we didn't see anything unusual. I'm sorry."

Didn't see anything unusual; what isn't unusual about this?

Mom's waiting up, as she always is. No matter where I go or who I'm with, mom's always waiting up.

She can see from our expressions and our multiplying manila envelope stack that nothing's new. Without saying a word I crawl onto my mattress and pull my blanket over my head. Also silent, my mom crawls onto my sister's mattress next to me and holds me.

Our sleeping arrangements have been a little unorthodox lately. My mattress has been moved out into the middle of the living room. My sister is sleeping in my parents' bed. Her mattress is also in the living room, right next to mine. My dad sleeps in his bed, but my mom sleeps on my sister's, next to mine in the living room. I'm guessing houses don't usually function like that. I know ours never did.

Ours was nothing like this. We were two loving parents, two beautiful, straight "A" athletic daughters, and two crazy dogs. *How could our normal, great life turn so upside down?*

I know how. I ruined it.

I ruined it by getting this pain.

Chapter Two

Notre Dame, my dream high school. I had wanted to go there my whole life and because it is a private school, it was really hard to get in. I worked my butt off to try to get in there. I called people from my past, and what was at the time my present. I asked them to write letters of recommendation for me. It was embarrassing and I felt like I was being a bother, but I did it anyway. I needed to get in.

The letters people wrote were beautiful and I still have them. I was called *impressive, intelligent, confident, centered, outgoing, focused, loving, real,* etc. I never really knew how much people thought of me until those letters. I never noticed the pride in their eyes when they introduced me to someone from their lives, or the support they gave me when I was struggling. The most humbling part that I took from all of those letters was that these were all well-liked, accomplished adults saying such nice things about me. They took time out of their lives to help me out, and at the same time made me realize how lucky I was. I felt honored and pleased with myself.

Having those closest to me sum me up was a very interesting experience. The kind words made me smile and the hopefulness of the letters got me excited. I was thrilled because everyone had such high expectations for me and my future, but that also made me nervous.

My dear friend Gay wrote:

> *...Even though this young woman has many talents that lead to almost endless possibilities for her future, the most important is that she is a truly lovely, kind, generous person. I've seen her relate to a 90-year-old man and a small child, kittens and dogs, kids her own age. She seems to have a special way with each. While every school wants talented, bright students like Georgia Huston, they really need great souls who will be a joy to teach*

and who will appreciate what they are given. Georgia is the kind of person who will not only take and absorb, but also will create and give back...

Confidence boost? Yeah, I would think so.

I had always been an athlete, ever since kindergarten, despite my serious asthma. My mom signed me up for T-Ball and that was it. I played year round, alternating between soccer, basketball, and baseball. At age 12, I was the only girl to "graduate" from Sherman Oaks Little League. I wasn't just the only girl on the team for most of those years, I was the only girl in my league.

I would play a soccer tournament in Santa Barbara, three games a day, and then race across town for basketball practice or baseball tryouts. I worked hard on my all-star teams, private lessons with professional players, tournament teams, and even off-season. It was a lot, but I loved it. I became an expert at holding my nose in stinky park bathrooms and skillful at changing uniforms in a moving car filled with the rest of my family.

Besides being an athlete, I was a great student. Ever since elementary school I had been a mediocre test taker, but my creativity shined through my reports and essays. I wasn't a bookworm like my younger sister, Veronica, but I did well.

I was also a performer. I'd been in my school choir throughout elementary school and when I moved up to Millikan Middle School I got into the Performing Arts Academy, where I took dance. I was in the chorus and several school musicals and was immersed in that world for a while.

The summer after sixth grade, I was a member of the cast of the touring "Joseph and the Amazing Technicolor Dreamcoat," at the Pantages Theatre in Hollywood. I was in the children's chorus, and I was on stage the whole show; even more than the leads. I was sitting with a group of other kids on the side of the stage, in costume, singing and dancing along with the stars. It was an amazing experience that I wouldn't trade for the world. Some people work their whole lives to perform on a stage like that. It was never my dream before then, and it especially hasn't been my dream since. That is not my calling, but I loved every minute of it.

I did that show for two weeks, twelve performances, and got paid more than I could have imagined.

During those same two weeks, my baseball team was in the playoffs. We won the championship of our league, undefeated and merciless. That meant that we moved on to the Tournament of Champions, a tournament of all the champion teams in the San Fernando Valley competing against each other. After school I would race across town to various fields and play in my baseball games, and then I would race into downtown Hollywood to perform at night. We ended up dominating that tournament and winning the whole thing. My name is still on a billboard at the Little League.

When I was in eighth grade, I was practicing basketball in my backyard. We had a hoop and a pretty big area to run around in. I was alone, shooting and doing lay-ups. I was running, doing a lay-up, when I rolled my right ankle and fell. I screamed for someone to help me. My sister Veronica came out and then immediately got my mom. I couldn't move for a long time. I'd had injuries throughout my life; everyone knows that's part of being an athlete. I'd had sprains and stitches, but nothing like this. I knew this one was different.

My dad was out of town, so my mom and sister did their best to get me into the car, ice pack in hand. We knew how long an ER would take, so we tried a Child Urgent Care place. They took me in right away and had me X-rayed.

It turned out I'd torn a couple of ligaments in my ankle. They put a brace on it and gave me crutches. That was the first time I was told to use crutches. They took a while to get used to.

The man I'll call Doctor One told me to stay home from school the next day, so I did. By that afternoon I was feeling a lot better, so I told my mom I wanted to go on a walk. She told me that probably wasn't a good idea on the crutches, but I insisted. So, she saddled up our twin huskies and we were off. It was great to get out of the house and it was a beautiful day. My mom kept telling me that we should probably head back, but I kept saying I wanted to go farther.

We got pretty far from the house and I was absolutely exhausted. We started back, but I didn't make it. I'd pushed myself too much. I sat on a stranger's lawn with my dogs, Spot and Striker, while my mom ran back to get the car.

At school I got teased for getting hurt playing a sport by myself, but hey, you only need yourself to hurt yourself. I couldn't dance for a couple of weeks or play sports, but I still went to all the dance classes and sports games to support my friends. In addition to the crutches, I was put in a special therapeutic boot that I could pump up to add pressure. Also, for the first time, I had to go to physical therapy. I didn't like my physical therapist that much, but my sports doctor, Dr. Two, sent me there; so I went. It was long and rough, but I healed and got right back into the swing of things.

> Dear Georgia Huston and Parents,
> Congratulations! I am pleased to inform you that you have been accepted as a member of Notre Dame's Class of 2012. Notre Dame is a school that offers…

I made it.

Chapter Three

Notre Dame was the most amazing school I had ever seen. I'd gone to public schools my whole life, and they are quite different. This place had sensor-motion faucets, touch-screen computer white-boards, and in the cafeteria you used your fingerprint to access your money account. I didn't go in knowing many people, but I made plenty of new friends. It was awesome.

By this point I had dropped basketball and moved from baseball to softball. I planned on playing soccer and softball in high school. My friend Marisa and I tried out for the soccer team freshman year. That tryout was quite a wake-up call; this wasn't AYSO anymore. These girls were serious and really, really good.

I didn't feel very confident. There were a lot of people trying out and not a lot of spots, but that Friday my name was on the list. Marisa and I were on the Junior Varsity Notre Dame soccer team. I was on top of the world.

The next nine weeks were the most physically challenging weeks I had ever faced. I pushed myself harder than I had ever before. It was serious physical conditioning, and like I said, this was no little kid league. After school we did wind sprints up and down the football field, we jump-roped, did weight training, long distance two-mile runs, everything. On those two-mile runs, we had to clock in under a certain time or we had to do extra step-ups on the bleachers after practice. I never had to do that, even with my asthma.

I was in the best shape of my life, but I also made so many more friends. I was a part of something and felt a strong sense of community among those girls. Also, during the training season, Marisa and I were playing on another park team and practicing with a club team. We had a lot on our plates, but loved every second of it.

I was going to the mall after school, football games on Fridays, and movies on the weekends. I was so happy and living the teenage life to the fullest. Boys were flirting with me, dresses started fitting me the way they were supposed to, and I was having slumber parties with friends. It was a whole new world.

I will never forget the first night I had this new kind of pain. It was different. I was at soccer practice at the Van Nuys-Sherman Oaks park. It was after dark and really cold. We were all in sweats and jackets, shivering our way through a drill, when a pain shot up the outside of my right leg. I kept playing, but after a while I had to stop. My coach was very understanding and the girls were sympathetic. They knew I wouldn't quit unless I really had to.

The pain stopped that night, and for a couple of days after. We thought it had vanished just as mysteriously as it had come, but it started bothering me again the next week. To this day, the only way I can really describe the feeling is that it was like a lightning bolt shooting up my leg.

That pain really restricted me, and soon after that my lower back started bothering me. This felt different though; it was more concentrated and felt like a constant pressure in the middle of my lower spine. It was actually really low, almost to my butt.

My mom stayed up late with me, icing my leg and massaging my back, but none of it seemed to do any good. I had a follow up appointment with Dr. Two to discuss my ankle, so my dad mentioned the leg pain I'd been complaining about. Dr. Two was concerned by this, so she ordered an MRI; my first of many.

They gave me a little locker and had me change into one of their great "gowns." I walked into the room and confronted a monster machine. I stared that little tube down. *Will I fit in there?* They had me put in earplugs and lie down. I had no idea what to expect, so I closed my eyes as they rolled me into the machine; my whole body was inside.

That machine makes the loudest noise ever, and it's right in your ears and all around you so it's a million times worse. I thought I could just sleep through the half hour MRI, but there's no way I could get used to the noise, because not only was it loud, it kept changing rhythms to keep me on my toes. When I decided to be adventurous I opened my eyes, only to immediately regret it. My nose was not even an inch away from the top; I was so close to the ceiling of the machine that my eyes couldn't even focus. That was my first and last time ever really feeling claustrophobic in those; I got used to it pretty fast after that.

That Friday we went back to Dr. Two's office. Her waiting room always took forever, even though there were not usually a lot of people in there; and it had the most boring channels on the TV so there wasn't anything to entertain you.

My dad and I walked into our assigned room and right away I noticed something was different. There was a mini-model of a spine on the counter. *She left it in here from her last patient.*

"Dr. Two will be with you as soon as possible."

"Okay, thank you," I said with a smile; this was before I knew what that really meant. This was before I lost faith.

A little later the doctor came in with my first set of manila envelopes.

"Hi Georgia, how are you?" she said pinning the MRIs onto the wall.

"I'm still having the pain. Yesterday was really bad. Did you find anything?"

"Yes, we did." I couldn't decide if this was good news or bad news. It was good because they found something so we could treat it and I would get better; it was bad because – well, they found something.

"On a scale of one to ten, where do you think your pain is?"

"Twelve."

"Do you know what a herniated disc is?" she asked, looking back and forth between me and my dad. He was standing next to the window. That's him, always standing.

"Georgia's cousin had a herniated disc," my dad mentioned. I hadn't even thought about that. My cousin Talia is a couple of years older than me, and she had surgery for a herniated disc not too long before. I'd never really asked her what exactly it was though.

"Well that's odd because it's not really hereditary," the doctor started, picking up the little model of a spine. She pointed at the bone areas. "These are vertebrae in the spine…"

Then she pointed at the sac-like ovals in between each vertebra. "These are intervertebral discs. They are soft and cushion each vertebra."

Her hand moved down the spine to a discolored, deformed disc. "This is a herniated disc. Notice the color and shape of the others, and then notice this one. Part of the disc is bulging out. The MRI showed that you have a herniated disc on your L5, which is in your lower back, right where your pain is. The part of the disc that is bulging out and slipping is compressing a nerve root and causing the pain in your right leg." She pointed at the MRI. "See, these are your other discs, all evenly colored and built. This one is your L5, do you understand?"

I nodded; my mind was blank. I heard what she was saying, but wasn't really listening. It was a lot to take in.

"Talia is not genetically related. She is technically a step cousin, so even if it was hereditary that wouldn't really be the case here," my dad informed the doctor. Even though Talia is my step cousin, she has been in my life since I was two. She is my family.

"Okay," Dr. Two smiled. "Then I guess it's just an incredible coincidence because this is extremely rare for children. What happened with Talia?"

"She had back surgery at fifteen. Is Georgia going to need surgery?" My dad's facial expression changed dramatically. Spinal surgery is not something to take lightly.

"That is an option," she said, pausing just long enough for me to feel the tension in the room. "We could have her start physical therapy and see how that works before we start seriously considering surgery. That's another option."

My dad turned and looked out the window. "Can we let you know later? I want to talk with my wife about this."

"Of course. Georgia, do you have any questions? You've been really quiet." She looked at me, putting down the model of a spine. But now it wasn't just a spine. It was my spine; a spine with a problem.

She was right, I hadn't really said anything. I guess I was just taking it all in. I didn't have any questions at the time, but I did have one request, "I want to change physical therapists."

Dr. Two laughed. "Yes, we can do that. So, if you don't have any questions, can I speak with your dad alone?"

I was surprised. *It's my body.* But I agreed and went out into the boring waiting room. I went to the water fountain and took a sip of the cold water. I felt it run down my throat, immediately relaxing me, and took a deep breath. *Herniated disc.*

I wondered what they were talking about in there. *Risks?*

A few minutes later my dad popped his head through the door and called me in. I put down the magazine and followed him into the second room on the right. Dr. Two was waiting for us.

"Hey Georgia, have a seat," she said motioning. I did. "Okay, so I talked to your dad" – *Oh really, is that why I left?* – "and we decided that it would be best if we give you some medication to help with the injury. I know you're already on Singular for your asthma, but this won't interfere with that at all." She scribbled something down and handed it to my dad, then looked back at me. "It's a type of steroid that I want you to take twice a day for two weeks, and then come in for your next appointment."

"Steroids? Will I get buff?" I asked, concerned.

She laughed, "No it will just help with the swelling. I gave your dad the number of a physical therapist who will take good care of you."

The doctor maintained strong eye contact with me. "Now with the pill, you might get what some people call 'roid rage.' Have you heard of that?"

I was confused. "Rage? Like I'm going to be aggressive?"

"Not necessarily, but possibly. I think you will just become extremely emotional and irritable. I'm telling you this ahead of time, so hopefully you will be able to notice the way you are acting, and change it to save your poor parents."

"I'll be fine," I said.

I think I would have more control over myself than a little pill.

I couldn't.

That little pill had so much power over me it was eye opening. That was the first time I'd taken anything stronger than an aspirin, and I wasn't prepared for what I was in for. Neither were my parents.

I was a wreck. Everything that was said to me was taken the wrong way and thrown back into the innocent speaker's face.

I remember one night my parents took me out for pizza, just the three of us; I don't remember where Veronica was. We went to a new place on Ventura Boulevard and I just started bawling for no reason in the middle of the restaurant. No matter what my parents said or how much I rationalized in my head, I couldn't stop crying.

So I learned how powerful a little pill could be; my first of many.

Chapter Four

My new physical therapist, Debra, was an absolute angel and the highlight of my days. She was a spunky lady who I could always make laugh. I told her things that I didn't tell many other people. Even though she was an adult, I felt like I could talk to her about anything. I told her about my crushes and which bands I liked. I even made her a mix-tape of the Jonas Brothers; that's how close we were. She saved me magazine articles and I would show her pictures of cute famous guys on the internet. She was and still is a very good friend of mine.

I looked forward to going there twice a week and working my hardest. Dr. Two had me quit my sports for the time being so we could get my herniated disc under control. It was hard for me, but I still stayed in touch with my teams and supported them at their games. Since I had always been an athlete, it was in me to always want to work out and exercise. I would like to say I was a good pupil of Debra's, but I don't know for sure. She would give me exercises to do at home, and I would always do them, if not more. *So, if I'm doing everything and beyond, then why am I still feeling this pain?*

By pure chance, my softball coach at the time was actually the head of orthopedic surgery at one of the leading hospitals in L.A. When my dad told him I wasn't going to be able to practice and why, he immediately said, "Bullshit. There's no way Georgia has a herniated disc."

At his request, we brought my MRIs to him one day after practice. He opened the envelope on the softball field and studied it. He reluctantly agreed that there was something there that could be interpreted as a herniated disc, but he wasn't persuaded.

"I don't believe she has a herniated disc."

"Yes I do," I said looking at the MRI like I actually knew what it was saying.

"I'm telling you your disc is fine."

"Then why am I having so much pain?" I snapped, getting irritated.
"I don't know, but it's not the disc."

I left there angry at Doctor Three because he didn't believe that I had a herniated disc. For some reason he was being stubborn and I didn't like that. I wasn't wrong; I couldn't be.

I was staying up late, alternating ice packs and heat packs, but after weeks and weeks I was still not back to playing with my soccer team. Notre Dame's season had already started and I hadn't played in a game yet. That was frustrating; doing all that work in conditioning, but not having played in a game. I showed up to every single practice after school, staying until eight-thirty, shivering like crazy, and I went to every single game, no matter how far away. I was the team's number one fan, which I enjoyed, but I wanted to be their number one forward. I wanted to score our goals and win our games.

We were getting worried about my continuing pain, so we decided to look to some other doctors for their ideas. The doctors who were suggested were surgeons. Surgery was the last thing any of us wanted to do, but it was starting to look like we had to go in that direction. The basic advice most people give is to get at least a second opinion, if not a third or more. We got more than that.

We made appointments with several doctors, visiting them multiple times. Because my cousin Talia had success with her herniated disc surgery, we began by asking her surgeon for help.

Dr. Four was a nice guy who looked at my MRIs and X-rays for a moment or two. *Dr. Four, be my hero.*

He examined and interviewed me. "On a scale of one to ten, where is your pain?"

"Twelve."

He said that he wanted to order another MRI, but from the people downstairs that he knew. So, we went down to their office. When we gave them the papers from Dr. Four there was of course another stack of forms we needed to fill out. The place was really crowded so my dad and I couldn't find seats next to each other. I filled out most of them and got up to hand the rest to my dad. When I got back, my seat was taken.

I went back to my dad to complain, but instead he gave me his phone and told me to call Notre Dame and tell them that I wouldn't be going to school that day. *Story of my life.*

"Hello, Notre Dame High School," the polite voice on the other side answered.

"Hi, Mrs. Harold. It's Georgia," I replied all too familiarly.

"Oh Georgia! I'll send you through to Mrs. Daniels."

"Thank you."

She knew why I was calling; she knew where to send me. I had to make far too many of these calls.

> *Where's the fire, what's the hurry about?*
> *You'd better cool it off before you burn it out.*
> *You've got so much to do and only so many hours in a day.*

But there is a fire, Billy. It runs down my leg and burns in my back. It started there, but now it's burning through everything else in its path; my sanity, my happiness, my hope – where does it end? I have way more things in my day than normal kids my age and I can't handle it. I'm not asking for more hours in a day, I just want the fire out. I can't handle this. I'm not strong enough.

I wasn't nervous at all; it was just an MRI, I knew what to do. I was a vet at this kind of stuff.

They gave me a gown and a locker and sent me on my way. When I got into the MRI room I sat down on the table, ready to go.

"Hello, Georgia. My name's Mike. Have you ever had an MRI before?" Mike asked as he walked in.

"Yes," I said.

"Okay great, so I'm just going to put the dye in and then we will be good to go." He took a needle out of a drawer. My heart stopped and I started to panic.

"What are you doing with that?!"

"I'm going to inject some of this purple dye into your bloodstream so we'll be able to see everything more clearly in the MRI." *Oh, my God.*

"They didn't do this with my last MRI," I argued.

"Dr. Four ordered this one – with contrast."

Anyone who knows me knows that I am the biggest baby ever when it comes to needles. I still have my mommy hold my hand and I turn my head away when I get shots at my checkups. But mommy wasn't there that day, and my dad just laughs at me whenever I ask him. I was on my own for this one. That was becoming a recurring theme with me.

The next day I had my first appointment with Dr. Five – an acupuncturist. Even though I am scared to death of any type of needle; thin or thick, tall or small, many people we know swear by acupuncture. The fact that I went, fighting my biggest fear, should illustrate how desperate I was for some pain relief.

Dr. Five was a polite, shy man. That being said, I got him out of his bubble on occasion. I was good at that, making people comfortable.

"Do they hurt? Tell me the truth, I don't like liars," I said, raising my eyebrows at the man prepping to stab me multiple times.

Dr. Five smiled, "If it hurt, why would so many people go to acupuncturists?"

"I don't like needles, doctor," I stated.

He laughed, "Not many people do."

When he was ready, he dimmed the lights and asked me to lie on my belly.

"So on a scale of one to ten, where is your pain?"

"Twelve."

"Twelve," he muttered to himself under his breath.

"Can I listen to my iPod?" I asked. He nodded.

He waited until I was ready, until I got my Billy Joel on. I closed my eyes and tried to focus on Billy's voice and not the situation at hand.

"Ah!" I squealed.

"I haven't even put a needle in yet, I was just rolling up your pants leg," Dr. Five said smugly.

"Well, then you poked me," I said, trying to figure out a cover.

The needles didn't really hurt, but if I moved or tensed up they hurt like crazy. In a way they forced me to stay relaxed, because they would hurt me if I wasn't. When I left Dr. Five's office I did feel better, a lot better; but by the time I got home the pain was back. Temporary relief was appreciated, but it simply wasn't enough. I needed a solution and every day that went by when I didn't get one, sunk me further and further into my depression.

Anyone with pain knows what I'm talking about. It is absolutely the most maddening and devastating thing ever, when you think you are better and then the pain comes back.

Everyone knows that they cannot control anyone else in the world but themselves; like when you're little and you tattle-tale on someone and the teacher or your parent says, "Why don't you just worry about yourself?" That's all I was trying to do here, worry about myself. If I didn't have any control over myself, *what could I control?* I was useless and I knew it, but there was nothing I could do about it.

Who's next?

If you were to think of what a doctor's office would look like in the future, that's Dr. Six's office. It had waterfalls coming down the walls and the biggest, clearest televisions I had ever seen in my life. The fish tanks were taller than I was and the fish were exotic and extremely colorful. He didn't have chairs in the waiting room; he had couches that looked like they should be in a movie star's living room. If there was an "MTV Cribs" for doctors' offices, he would be on it.

Dr. Six wasn't a pediatric specialist but he was a highly regarded orthopedic surgeon. After I filled out my packet of where the pain was, how long it had been there, and how bad it was, we only had to wait about ten minutes; *I like this guy already.* We never got in to see anyone that fast.

We followed the nurse into our room, but it wasn't really an exam room – it was more like a luxury suite. When Dr. Six came in I was so excited; *he had to be good to have such an impressive office.*

"Hello, I'm Dr. Six," he said shaking my dad's hand first, then mine.

"I'm Jimmy, this is Georgia," my dad said.

"So you have severe back pain?"

"And leg pain," I added.

"Right, and leg pain," he said as he read my chart. "If ten is the worst pain possible and one is no pain at all, where is your pain on that scale?"

"Twelve."

"These are her MRIs and a few X-rays," my dad said, showing the stack of manila envelopes like evidence in a court case we couldn't win.

"Okay, I'll take a look and I'll be right back," and he was gone.

When he came back, he had a few of the MRI films in his hand and the rest in the envelope. He put the envelope down, but still kept those pages in his hand. *Dr. Six, be my hero.*

"I took a closer look, and she does not have a herniated disc," he said holding up the MRIs so we could see them. *Umm, yes I do.*

"From these MRIs, I can see how someone could think they saw a herniated disc on the L5. But, the technician took it from the wrong angle, elongating the shape of the disc and making it look deformed, when in fact it's merely the perspective of the image."

"So what does this mean?" my dad asked.

"Georgia does not have a herniated disc," he answered but didn't seem that relieved.

"Then what's causing her pain?"

"The problem is not in her back," he said.

He had a really cocky attitude, but then so do most doctors, especially surgeons. I was learning that doctors are egotistical and all think they are the best. "Stand up for me."

He started doing the usual probing up and down the side of my left leg, and then my right; then the inside of both. "Is your pain around here?" he asked, his hand right where my pain always was.

"Yeah, how'd you know?" My heart skipped a beat; *he found it.*

"I think you have what is called bursitis. That is when a bursa in your body, in this case your leg, gets inflamed. A bursa is a sac filled with fluid that cushions some of your joints. That's this little lump right here," he said tapping my leg.

I put my hand where his was. "I can barely feel anything."

My dad came over to feel. "Are you sure that's what it is?"

"Yes," Dr. Six nodded. "Extremely sure."

"So what do we do about the bursitis?" my dad asked, still feeling around my leg to try to find what Dr. Six found.

"The thing to do with bursitis is to inject steroids into the inflamed area," he said so matter-of-factly that I was stunned. *Steroids, again?*

"You mean like a shot?" I asked, panicking. "I don't do shots."

"Yes, a shot. But it won't hurt," he answered, obviously not realizing how uneasy that made me.

"What are the side effects?" my dad asked.

"Well, the shot will make the bursa really hard and bulge out a little bit," he said like it was nothing.

"How long will that last?"

"It will be permanent, but she won't have any more pain."

My jaw dropped.

"And what if it doesn't work?" my dad persisted. "What if the pain doesn't stop?"

"Oh, that won't happen," Dr. Six stated. He seemed offended by my dad's question.

"But what if?"

"Then she'll still have the hard bump that I told you about." *Oh, hell, no.*

"What are our other options?" My dad wasn't going to let me be injected and create a deformity.

Dr. Six relented. "We can try some medicine. That might help." *More pills.* "And I'll give you something for pain, too."

We went home that night empty handed. Again. We'd had an answer; *where'd it go?*

"What do you mean? Not a herniated disc?" My mom was wide-eyed. I put the blanket over my head while I plopped down onto their big king-sized bed.

"They took the MRI wrong," my dad explained, sitting on the couch and putting the TV on mute.

"So then what does she have?"

One of my two dogs, Spot or Striker, stuck her nose under my blanket. I didn't know which dog it was because I only saw the nose and they're twins. I pushed her away, but as soon as I did, I regretted it. My dogs always knew when I needed a hug or just some attention. Whenever I'm crying, one of them always seems to find me and rub up against me until I pet her. That's what one of them was trying to do then, but I pushed her away. I had a way of doing that, pushing away people who were trying to help me.

"We don't know," my dad said, looking at the wall.

"What do we do now?" my mom asked, sliding off the chair onto the floor.

My dad thought about it. "We should call Debra first thing in the morning and tell her what's going on. I guess we don't need to go to physical therapy anymore."

That made me sad. I loved Debra. *What was I going to do without my Jonas Brothers buddy?*

"So all that money and time chasing the herniated disc was a waste?" my mom asked.

"Lynn, please don't."

"Why did Dr. Two say she had a herniated disc?" She was so frustrated.

"I told you it was the technician," he repeated, trying to calm her down. "Lynn, please don't think about the money right now, let's just try to figure this out."

"When's the appointment with Dr. Seven?" My mom sat on the chair next to the couch. She looked so defeated. That's what this does to you; it defeats you. It makes you question everything, *what are we doing wrong?*

"It's on Wednesday."

That was the last thing I heard before I fell asleep. They probably thought I knocked out before that, but I didn't. As I drifted off, different thoughts went through my mind. I forgot about my biology homework.

Uh oh. I'll do it during lunch tomorrow. Thank God that's my seventh period. I also thought about how I was going to be missing algebra on Wednesday for my appointment with Dr. Seven. At least I have an "A" in that class. I forgot to call Solene about hanging out on Saturday. I'll do that later....

Now up, Dr. Seven.

"Georgia," the receptionist called from her desk, "first door on the right." The room was really small but my dad and I fit; I was still in my school uniform, which is the case for most of my doctors' appointments at this time.

There was a knock at the door almost immediately and in walked a little man with white hair and glasses; a lot older than I had expected. He was cute though and I remember he was wearing a "Winnie the Pooh" tie that made me smile.

"Hi, I'm Dr. Seven," he said shaking my hand and then my dad's.

"Jimmy," my dad said with a hint of a smile.

"I'm Georgia," I said.

"So what seems to be the problem here?" he asked, sitting down in the chair across from my dad. He was a highly regarded pediatric orthopedic surgeon who had helped people we knew. A specialist.

We told him that I had a herniated disc and that physical therapy hadn't been helping, so we wanted his diagnosis. My dad handed him my envelope of MRIs, which Dr. Seven flipped through one by one to examine. After looking at them for a couple of minutes, he said he wanted to look at them more closely in his office. *Dr. Seven, be my hero.*

When he came back, he put the MRIs down on a chair and came over to me. "Where's your pain, on a scale of one to ten, ten being the worst pain possible."

"Then my pain's a twelve."

"Can you turn around for me?"

I obeyed. He ran his fingers up and down my spine, pressing in certain areas, trying to find my sensitive spots. He had me lie down on my back and he took a tape measure out of his pocket. *What?*

Dr. Seven held one end of the tape at my big toe on my left foot and then brought it up my leg to where my skort ended. He took out a black marker and started drawing lines up and down my leg, following the tape measure. I looked at my dad, who had the same puzzled expression.

"I found the problem," he said after not even a full minute. He put his tape measure back into his pocket. "Your left leg is longer than your right." He seemed so content with his diagnosis.

I could tell my dad wasn't buying it. "How much longer is it?" he asked, extremely skeptical.

"The difference is about a quarter of an inch," Dr. Seven said, while writing something in a notebook.

"So the reason she is up late at night crying in pain is that there's a quarter of an inch difference in her leg lengths?"

"Yes."

"So what do we do about this?" My dad was ready to try anything.

"I'm going to write you a prescription right now – for a lift to put in your shoe." *Is he serious?*

"Is that really going to solve the problem?" my dad asked.

"Yes, because the legs are the foundation for all of her balance. If they're not at the same length, her whole body is going to be in a funk."

"So," my dad said, holding up the prescription for my lift, "this will stop her pain?"

"Try that."

When we got home my dad held up the little cork pad that we'd gotten from a shoe repair shop – it was a quarter of an inch thick. "He said this will help."

I crawled into my parents' bed and covered my face with a blanket. *Nobody can see me.*

"What is that?" my sister Veronica asked, peering out from behind her book. She's the only person I know who will take books to her friends' swimming parties and to movie theatres. She's always been like that.

"It's a lift for Georgia's shoe," dad said, not fully confident with his next statement. "Dr. Seven said this will help her pain."

"Don't go home," Raquel pleaded with me. "You're halfway through the day. Stick it out for two more classes."

"I can't," I said, sitting down on a bench. "It's really bad."

"You went home Friday, too," she said.

"I was hurting Friday, too," I argued.

"Seriously George, don't go home."

I had to. I crawled into my parents' bed and clicked the TV on. That's where I spent most of my time; in the dark, bundled under a huge blanket. Even though the TV was on, I didn't even watch it. It's just always on in the background; it's comforting to me. I grabbed my notebook and pencil and started sketching. That's what I always did when I was sad, angry, upset, happy, anything; it always helped.

Drawing calmed me down and made everything better. It was incredible to me how each little line comes together and makes something recognizable, something that's just yours. It doesn't always come out exactly the way you pictured it. Sometimes it comes out completely different, but sometimes it comes out even better.

I loved testing the boundaries and drawing things that most people wouldn't think of drawing. If you were to flip through my sketchbook at the time you would have seen feet, hands, girls putting on nail polish, and ceiling fans. I would use mirrors to draw. I would put myself in odd poses, like putting on a pair of jeans, and I would draw. I wouldn't use the mirrors necessarily to make the picture look like me, but to just have a better idea of what a body would look like; the proportions and the curves. I was a perfectionist when it came to my art and wouldn't even show a drawing to my parents if I didn't think it was great.

But I didn't make my art to show people. My closest friends didn't even know I was an artist. I was honestly embarrassed about my art. When people would come over and my dad would want me to show them some of my drawings, I would refuse. It was so personal to me, I didn't think anyone else would understand. I was wrong though; art turned out to be my only way of communicating with the world.

As my good friend Andy wrote me recently:

Keep making art.
When everything else fails you, it will be your savior.
I speak from experience.

There is a sense of community among all artists that I appreciate. I have learned that it doesn't matter if you are a writer, a photographer, a painter, anything; we all have our own way of sharing how we are feeling with the outside world, and they are all special.

Dr. Four had been the one to order the MRIs, but on our next visit he flipped through them quickly and returned them to my dad. We both noticed that Dr. Four never looked at the technician's written report before giving up on me. Later my dad read it and wondered what it meant by "possible pars defect."

Chapter Five

The medicine from Dr. Six didn't help.

"I need more information. I can send you to get a bone scan and see if that shows us anything," Dr. Six offered.

"Okay," my dad seemed relieved. "Let's do that."

"If you go to Tarzana hospital," he said writing something on his pad, "they will take you in right away. I'll call ahead."

"Great," my dad said, taking the prescription. "Thank you."

When we got to the hospital the security guard showed us where to go. It was a really small room in the middle of a hallway that had two windows on opposite sides of the room. We went to the wrong window at first, but then the correct one gave us the paperwork to fill out. I wished I could just save all my information on my laptop and hand that to everyone so I wouldn't have to keep rewriting it a million times.

"What's Apateece's work number?" I asked my dad. As long as I could remember I had always put my uncle Steve as my emergency contact. When I was little I couldn't say "Uncle Steve," so I substituted "Apateece." The name stuck.

"Here," my dad said, handing me his phone.

When I was done I brought the papers back to the window. The lady looked ticked off. "No, you get them from this window, but you return them to that one."

"Oh, sorry." *Someone's having a bad day.*

I'm not usually claustrophobic, but for some reason I always am in hospitals, ever since all this started and I practically lived in hospitals. Even though they are not small rooms, the never-ending off-white walls and meaningless pictures of landscapes make my throat close up and my thoughts jumble. Hospital corridors seem to go forever yet I feel trapped.

"Georgia Huston?" My dad and I got up. No stranger ever pronounces my last name correctly. It's spelled "Huston," but it's pronounced like the city "Houston." But I don't correct them; *what's the point?* I'm never going to see them again anyway. Sometimes I just cut to the chase and say my name is "Huston," saying it wrong on purpose. It saves them from searching for me under "H-o."

The lady in scrubs took me into a room and had me sit down. She started to tie a blue band around my arm and took out a syringe. I pulled my arm away at the exact time she pulled the cap off of the needle.

"What are you doing?!"

"Oh this?" she held up the needle. "This is just blue dye."

"You have the wrong person, my last name is Huston." I took off the blue rubber tie.

She looked at her folder. "Right, Georgia."

"What exactly does it say I'm here for?" I asked, getting up and peering over her shoulder to see my papers.

"It says that Dr. Six ordered you a bone scan for today."

"He did. I know that."

"So let me tie this back on your arm," she said, picking up the blue tie from the table.

I remained standing. "My dad said a bone scan is like an X-ray." My memory shot back to the purple dye that Mike shot into me for my last MRI. *Ugh.*

After the shot, she said that I should drink plenty of liquids for the next hour or they would have to inject more of the dye. So my dad and I went to a really great Mexican restaurant, *Las Fuentes,* where I spotted a familiar face.

"Jerry!" I called to him.

We had lunch that day with one of my former softball coaches. We told him about what we had been going through and how difficult it had been. He sympathized, but had no idea.

That was one of the many frustrations about all of this. No one truly understood. You could tell them every last detail of the past year or so and it would sound terrible, but it would never sound as bad as it really was.

I fell asleep during the bone scan, like I'd been knocked out cold. It was great. She put a blanket on me. It wasn't loud like an MRI and I didn't have to move around like with X-rays. I could just relax and drift off while the machine traced my newly blue blood.

"Mows!" My two-year-old cousin, Sarah, always called my dogs "mows." She couldn't say the word "animals," so she invented the word "mows."

"Hi Sare-Sare," my mom said, picking her up and giving her a hug.

"Hey Dawn," I called, hugging her and then Apateece.

"Hi Georgia, how are you doing?" Aunt Dawn asked, putting down Sarah's diaper bag.

"Not great."

"Aw, I'm so sorry," she said making a sad face.

"Jaja!" Sarah said, grabbing my leg. She called me "Jaja," my sister "Nakka," my dad "Immy," and my mom "Auntie Nin." We still use those names for each other.

"Hello Sarah," I said smiling.

"Pick me up!" she said, jumping up and down with her arms in the air. I bent down and lifted her – immediately the horrible pain started pulsating in my back. I winced and put Sarah down.

"Pick me up!"

"I can't, Sare. I'm sorry," I said, visibly defeated as I sat down on the couch.

"Why?" She looked up at me with her big blue eyes.

"Because my back hurts."

"Like Taya?"

"Yes, just like Talia."

> *But you know that when the truth is told...*
> *That you can get what you want or you can just get old.*
> *You're gonna kick off before you even get halfway*
> *through*
> *When will you realize, Vienna waits for you?*

That's all that's going to happen to me, I'm just going to get old. Even though my life is on pause, time is still going and the clock is still running. No one is waiting for me, I will never catch up. I will never be able to go to my freshman Homecoming dance, I will never be able to go to Solene's fifteenth birthday party; all of that is in the past – done. Even though my life is stopped, it seems like everyone else's is on fast forward.

The best part about Billy's lyrics, "Vienna waits for you." Vienna can signify any place, real or fictional or even just a state of mind; Vienna can be anywhere you want it to be. It is somewhere that you want to go without even knowing that you want to go there. The great part is that this magical place has no time limit, Vienna will always be there for you and when you're ready, it's ready; Vienna's waiting.

For a few weeks we bounced between doctors, guided by my life-long physician, Dr. Eight. All of these doctors knew one another and were very respectful, but sometimes we saw hints of raised eyebrows as another doctor's diagnosis was discussed. This was all outside of Dr. Eight's specialty, but she mentioned that if I didn't get relief, we could apply to the UCLA Pediatric Pain Management Clinic. We thought that sounded too desperate.

We brought the bone scans and the MRIs back to Dr. Six.
"Okay," he said looking up at me, "it's not bursitis."
Oh my gosh, thank God my dad didn't let him give me that permanent deforming shot.
"So what is it?" I asked. If he knew it wasn't that, he must see something else.
"I don't know, I don't see anything wrong with your films. Is your pain still a twelve?" he asked.
I nodded.
"There's nothing I can find that is wrong with you," he answered. "I can't help you."
Nothing wrong with me?
"If there is nothing wrong, then why is she feeling like this?" my dad asked, clearly irritated.
"I don't know, I just don't." He walked over to the window and looked out for a moment. The lightning pain shot down my right leg and I winced, but no one saw. "I'm going to refer you to someone, Dr. Nine. If anyone will know, it's him."
Okay, at least he is trying to help. I thought that before I knew what referrals really meant. They are a polite way of saying, "Hey, I give up, so now you're someone else's problem." That's all they are.
We called Dr. Nine's office while we were in the elevator leaving Dr. Six; the sooner you make the appointment, the sooner you see the doctor. They said that it was their lunch break, but still asked, "How soon can you get here?"

My dad's eyebrow went up, "We can be there in fifteen minutes."

"Then come now."

This guy was going to be different, I could feel it. *He's willing to see me during his lunch break?*

Dr. Nine's office was in the ghetto. I had never been to this area of Los Angeles before, and I could see why. We parked the car and walked across the street into an old building from the sixties. It was only three stories high, but the architecture made it look massive. There were huge dark brown block-like structures hanging from the walls, and the glass sliding doors had graffiti scribed into them.

I hate elevators, so obviously going into an old creaky one with a few light bulbs out wasn't fun for me. I still remember his elevator. The buttons had to be pressed multiple times and with more force than usual. The doors would close and then you would have to wait before you shakily moved upwards. Dr. Nine was on the third floor at the end of the first hallway. Some areas of the third level were dark because lights were out. It was seriously something out of a horror movie.

We opened the creaky door and entered the dimly lit waiting room. "Kung Fu Panda" was playing on the small box TV. It was stuffy and the couches looked like they were picked off the street after a family had dumped them on the curb. The room desperately needed some air freshener and the toys were dirty and old. The waiting room was completely empty which surprised me until I remembered it was their lunch break. Everything about this place was super sketchy.

"Okay Georgia, come on in." That was the first time I had ever been called in right away, so I left the baby-blue paint-chipping walls of the waiting room and went into a long hallway. On the faded white walls were extremely dated murals of "Winnie the Pooh." You could tell they were old by the worn out colors and the style of the characters.

The nurse walking us to the exam room asked if I wanted lemonade or cookies as we passed a table with a tray full of both. I took a cup of lemonade, but wondered why they had so many snacks if no one was there.

"This is your room. Dr. Nine will be with you as soon as possible," the nurse said, motioning to the room to our left. The room looked like everything else in the office. There were blinds missing from the window and cracks in the walls.

"Quite a place isn't it?" My dad laughed.

"Kind of scary," I said, looking around.

"We'll try anything."

"I know, dad." *How could someone as successful as Dr. Six send us to a dump like this?*

A few minutes went by and two nurses came in asking various questions; taking my temperature, blood pressure, etc. All the nurses, male and female, were young and happy people who seemed to enjoy working there. They all spoke so highly of Dr. Nine. I will never forget how much everyone there loved him and thought he was the best. They said he was a caring man who put patients first. He was on-call twenty-four/seven. I think that said a lot about his intentions.

My dad and I were waiting silently when we heard a really odd sound. It was like a scratching and grinding sound getting louder and louder. I couldn't place the sound for the life of me. Then, in he walks. *This is the famous Dr. Nine?*

He looked older than my grandpa and he was shorter than me because he was hunched over so far. He had the thickest glasses I have ever seen and was walking with a cane; his foot was in a boot like he'd injured it. He wasn't exactly what I was expecting, but what do I know?

He was followed by a male nurse I'd seen earlier, who helped him around the room and held papers for him. Dr. Nine didn't make eye contact with my dad or me until after talking to us for probably ten minutes. He puzzled me. Even though he rarely made eye contact at all, you could always tell he was listening intently and carefully thinking at the same time. He scribbled lots and lots of notes.

"Hi Georgia," he said looking down at his papers. "It says here you have some back and leg pain."

"That's correct," I politely answered.

"Lower back pain," he said, not really to anyone in the room, just to himself. He was reading my file. "You were told it was a herniated disc, then that it wasn't. The same with bursitis. Now you're thinking that it's because your legs make you off balanced." He finally looked up at me. That was the first time I looked into his eyes and saw how tired, but determined, he looked. *Dr. Nine, be my hero.*

"Here are her MRIs, but Dr. Six told us they are taken at a bad angle," my dad said, handing him the manila envelopes.

"Oh, Dr. Six," he said under his breath, he seemed pleased. He took one out of the envelope and stared at it for a long time. He examined each centimeter of it with such determination and effort that I was thoroughly impressed. He took that much care with each of my films.

He left and went into his office for a little bit. When he came back he said that he might have found something, but didn't want to tell us until he was sure. "I want to take more X-rays of your back."

"Andrew here," he pointed to the nurse, "will take you to get X-rayed." And that was it. He left. He was a really odd man.

I was led into the back and told to lie down on a table. I remember the guys taking my X-rays were really funny and nice. They put me at ease.

When Dr. Nine came in with the X-rays, I felt so hopeful. He had to know what was happening; *he's going to find it on the X-ray!*

"On a scale of ten to one, one being no pain and ten being the worst, where is your pain?"

"It's a twelve."

"All the time?" He raised an eyebrow.

"Yes, all the time."

"Stand up for me please," he said, taking off his glasses. I stood up and he had me turn away from him. He ran his fingers up and down my spine and I told him where it hurt – my lower back as usual. "You can sit back down."

"Well," he started. *Just spit it out already!* "You have a..." and then he muttered something.

What?

Dr. Nine mumbled some single half-heard technical word.

My dad spoke for both of us. "What did you say?"

He mumbled again.

I looked at my dad. He couldn't understand it either, but he stopped asking. Later we would learn that the word was "spondylolysis."

We'd learn that it's also known as a pars defect. *Like that helps.*

"It's common in adolescent athletes who overtrain, and I see it on your lumbar vertebrae, L5," Dr. Nine said, pointing at one of my new X-rays.

My dad and I had no idea what we were looking at.

"So what does this mean?" my dad asked. For some reason I was always really quiet at my appointments.

"It's a stress fracture," he started.

"A fracture?" I interrupted, "Is my back broken?"

The doctor looked at me. "Technically speaking, yes. It is a defect of a vertebra and is most commonly found at the L5, which is where yours is. The two bump-like things on top of that vertebra, right here, are fractured. It says that on one of the MRI reports, I wonder why nobody saw it. How many doctors looked at these?" *Uh oh.*

"A lot. Is this why she's having pain?" my dad asked.

"Well, I suspect this is the reason, but the interesting thing about this is that about one out of ten people have it. They sometimes live their whole lives without knowing they have it, not feeling any pain. It's not unheard of for people to complain about it though. That's what we have here. It's bothering Georgia, so I'm going to send you to see some great people who will make you a cast. I'll call ahead so they know exactly how I want it."

He wrote something down, ripped it out of his notebook, and handed it to my dad. "Go see Paul, and then get back to me."

"We'll do that right away," my dad promised, folding the paper and putting it in his pocket.

"Wait," I said. "What kind of cast if it's my spine?"

"Well," he looked at me sympathetically, "it will be a body cast."

Body cast? I can't have a body cast! I had no idea what to expect or how much of my body it would cover, but I could tell already that it wouldn't be fun. Kids at school had better not be able to see it. *It'll be thin right? No one will be able to tell.*

When we left and were passing through the formerly empty waiting room, there were more people in there than could fit comfortably. There were many families and little kids running around. Dr. Nine's kindness was no secret.

Chapter Six

"Pars defect, huh," my grandpa repeated blankly.

"Yeah, he said that a lot of people have it, it just doesn't bother them," I explained.

"Then why does it bother you?" he asked.

"I don't know."

"How long until it's better?"

"I don't know, Grandpa." *I don't know, I don't know. Stop asking me questions that I don't have the answers to. I don't know!*

"I want to see you play softball at Notre Dame," he said.

"I know you do." I was clearly getting irritated. I had no control over any of this. My grandparents were die-hard Catholics and the fact that I, their un-religious granddaughter, was going to a Catholic school made them ecstatic.

Besides that, my grandpa just wanted to see me playing softball again. He was one of my biggest fans when it came to my baseball career. He loved the sport and loved watching me play it. He would drive hours on Saturdays to watch me play and it made me so happy to see him in his white sun hat up in the stands. I loved my grandpa.

"Oh, I almost forgot," he said standing up and walking to his closet. "I thought these might interest you."

I took the newspaper clippings from his hand and looked at them. There were three cartoons and two stories about successful kids.

"Thanks Grandpa," I said with a gentle smile. He would always save me random things from the newspaper and either mail them to me or wait until our next visit. I'm still puzzled about how some of the things reminded him of me, but I kept them all anyway.

"Peaches! Peaches, come here!" my mom shouted from the other room. She always calls me "Peaches," ever since I was a baby because of the "Georgia peaches." She also calls me "George," but so does everyone else.

37

My grandpa and I went into the other room. He and my grandma lived in an assisted living facility so they only had two rooms and one bathroom area to share. My mom and sister were out on the porch, while my grandma was sitting by the door in her wheelchair. She wasn't doing well.

They were all looking at the bird feeder that was hanging from a tree by the porch. There were a couple of hummingbirds on it. Hummingbirds were the only type of bird that could eat from their bird feeder because of their long, thin beaks. There were always hummingbirds around my grandparents' home, even at their old house. That's the reason I love hummingbirds so much, they remind me of my grandparents.

The next day we went to the orthopedic guy Dr. Nine referred us to. It was an okay office, definitely better than Dr. Nine's. You could tell a majority of his patients were children because of the atmosphere; colorful and exciting.

The technician who was going to make my cast was a middle-aged man named Paul. He was really nice and genuine. He was going to be the one to help me. *Paul, be my hero.*

I didn't spend a lot of time with him, but he was sympathetic and truly believed the cast would help me; *so it will.*

He sent me to a room and had me take off my clothes and put on a nylon stocking type thing that was big enough to fit my whole body. He came in with my dad and took measurements of the areas where he was going to be fitting the cast. *Wait, this can't be right. Why is he measuring my leg? The problem is in my back.*

He started to stick cold, goopy stuff all over my body until it hardened. When he thought it was hard enough, he took out a vibrating electric saw.

"What is that!" I asked, clearly alarmed.

"I'm going to cut you out of this," he said coming closer.

"Wait, wait. What happens when it cracks through? Am I going to get cut?"

"No," Paul laughed, "give me your finger."

When he brought the blade closer, I pulled away.

"What are you doing?!"

"It won't hurt, look," he said smiling, bringing the blade to his skin; no blood or cuts or anything.

I took a deep breath and gave him my hand. I winced when he brought the tool to my hand, but it didn't hurt. It actually tickled a little bit.

"If that can't cut through my skin, how is it going to cut through this hardened cast?" I asked.

"It will."

He was right; he cut right through that thing. That little blade will always be a mystery to me.

He told us the cast would be ready in about a week, so we made our next appointment and left. I will never forget the car ride home. It was the first time I was out of control. It was a preview of what was to come.

We were in the car and I suddenly felt blood rushing to my head. I was dizzy and my heart was beating very fast. I closed my eyes and opened the window, feeling the breeze come into the car, down my throat, and over my body. I couldn't focus on any thoughts, which really scared me. Although I frequently suffer from migraines, this was different. I didn't tell my dad how I was feeling. I thought I was just a little sick.

Soon these would be the warning symptoms for severe panic attacks, but I didn't know it at the time.

Solene gave me a strange look. "You broke your back?"

"Then how are you standing and walking?" Marisa wondered, looking at my back.

"It's like a fracture," I tried to explain, but I had no idea what I was talking about.

"When did you fracture it?" Marisa asked.

"I don't know," I answered.

"So you broke your back without even knowing it?" Raquel inquired, kind of laughing at me. "How do you do that?"

"It can't be broken," Solene argued. "Wouldn't you be paralyzed or something?"

"It's fractured, I don't know anything else." I just wanted the questions to stop.

"Are you going to go back to physical therapy?" Raquel asked.

"No, they're giving me a cast," I said unhappily.

"A cast! Where is it going to be?" Solene looked surprised.

"I don't know yet." *Stop asking me questions, please.*

"What about soccer? How long is the cast going to be on? The season ends in like a month," Marisa added, making everything worse.

"Seriously, I have no idea yet. You guys will be the first to know." I tried to drop it. The bell rang to save me; time for art class.

Ah, Mr. Lee's art class; a.k.a. my escape. I sat in my seat just long enough for him to tell us all to get up; we were going to be drawing outside today. My art class buddy, Braden, and I went out to look for a good spot to draw from. Mr. Lee said we could draw from anywhere on campus so Braden and I chose an area by the Lecture Hall. We sat on the concrete. *Thank God I didn't wear a khaki skirt today; my butt would be so dirty.*

Braden started drawing a palm tree from far away. I picked up my raw charcoal and blank notebook and started to draw a different tree. It was scrawny and not healthy at all, but I thought that would be a lot more interesting to draw than a live, flourishing plant. Everyone notices those, but not many people pay attention to the struggling ones.

It took me a while to decide what kind of style I wanted to draw it in. I could do it lightly and soft, the way the plant really looks; weak. But instead I decided to draw the suffering plant with bold, dark strokes. I wanted to use a completely different style than would be expected for such a plant. It may look weak from the outside, the insufficient leaves and the thin branches, but the strong style I was drawing with showed that it was in fact strong and fighting. Not everything is what it appears.

Mr. Lee put my picture up on the wall, as usual. He always put my art up on the walls, which is why I would only put my name on the back. Since it was usually the only student art that was up in the room, I was embarrassed. I don't know why I was embarrassed by my art, but I was, so my name was always hidden on the back.

After art class came religion class, Introduction to Catholicism. It was a mandatory class because it was a Catholic school. I had never been religious, so everything in that class was pretty new to me.

Ms. Loya would say over and over again, "God has a reason for everything." *Really? Then why is he making my life this difficult?*

Some people may say it's a challenge, that he's testing me; but I would say no. I would say that even if there is a God, which I have never been sure of, he was not testing me; he was torturing me. He was robbing me of precious time and experiences.

I missed going to the movies Friday because I had to get fitted for my cast. I couldn't have a sleepover at Jenny's on Saturday night because I was in so much pain I couldn't get out of bed. If God really does have a reason for everything, then God has some explaining to do.

Soccer practice that night was really long. It's hard to stay at school from seven-thirty a.m. to eight p.m. That's a long day, especially when you are watching other people doing the thing you love. But it's not only that I loved it, I deserved it.

When I got home I went straight into my parents' room, my comfort zone. I turned off the light and put the blanket over my head. To this day I always do that when I'm upset, cover my face with a blanket or towel. It makes me feel safe. I know it's immature to hide like that, but it relaxes me. I guess it's like when little kids close their eyes, or when they hide just their face, and think since they can't see you, you can't see them. It's a good strategy; if I couldn't see anything, I couldn't be seen. *Maybe since no one can see me, I'm invisible; and since I'm invisible, maybe the pain can't find me. Maybe.*

But somehow, no matter how many blankets I used to cover myself, the pain found me. I started to whimper as it crept back into my body. I tried to fight off the unwanted intruder but it insisted. I lay there helpless and alone while it took over my body. It started in my lower back and quickly traveled up my back and down my right leg at the same time.

My pain was like when you walk on the beach and you leave your footprints in the sand. If you turn around and look at your footprints, they show you where you've been and where you are now. But, when the waves of the ocean come up onto your footsteps, it washes them away. You can no longer tell where you came from, just where you are at the moment. My pain was like the unforgiving ocean, erasing all of my past. I could no longer tell where I came from or who I was. I could only lift up my feet and see the footprints I was making now. I didn't like where my footprints were.

I didn't want my past to be erased, I was happy with who I was. But, sometimes you don't have a choice with the direction your life is going to go in. I always thought I would be the only one defining my future, but I was wrong; and that scared me.

I broke down crying. This was my first time really having a meltdown about this whole thing; the stress was just too much. This pain wasn't just physically exhausting, it was emotionally draining.

My mind started racing but I couldn't think. It felt just like in the car on the way back from Paul's. My heart was beating out of my chest and I felt this strange tingling in my hands and feet. I was breathing faster than I ever had before; *this can't be an asthma attack, can it?*

I was so out of breath I couldn't even yell for my dad. I was thinking of ways to get his attention from across the house. I tried to get up, but I just collapsed onto the carpet. My feet were cramping and I yelped. I managed to get back on the bed and grabbed my phone. I pressed his number on my speed dial.

I heard it ringing in his office, "Hello?"

I didn't say anything, I couldn't. I was just panting and crying,

"Georgia?" *Yes! Get in here!*

When I didn't answer, I heard him get out of his chair. *What is happening?*

"What's wrong?" he asked desperately when he saw me shaking on his bed. I kept my eyes and mouth shut. *The world can't see me if I can't see it.* "Georgia, talk to me," he said sitting down next to me on the bed.

"I-I-I d-don't know," I stuttered under my breath.

"Calm down, Georgia, you're hyperventilating," he said.

Hyperventilating? What? I thought that was something that happens in extremely cold water, like on "Deadliest Catch."

"Listen to me, Georgia. You need to calm down."

"Wha-a-t-t-t is ha-happening t-to me?" I asked in between sobs. I couldn't move my hands.

"Lynn!" My dad yelled for my mom, but instead my sister came in.

"What's going on?" she asked, clearly horrified. Her eyes were wide as she watched me quivering uncontrollably on the bed.

"Get your mom," my dad said urgently, turning on the light.

"No! No, no! P-please turn that-t off," I pleaded.

"I'm gonna keep it on for a little bit," he answered.

"Oh my God! What happened?!" my mom cried out covering her mouth with her hand. She came onto the bed and held me.

"N-no no no-o-o," I begged, "Leav-ve me al-lon-ne." I didn't mean to hurt her feelings by pushing her away; I needed air. *Where did all the air go?*

My mom stood up and looked at my dad, tears in her eyes. "What's going on?!"

"I think she's having a panic attack," my dad said watching me carefully.

Panic attack?!

Chapter Seven

My dad sat down next to me. "Georgia, Georgia look at me." I turned my head. "You need to slow down your breathing...."

"I c-can't!" I snapped back at him.

"Georgia, you have to," he argued.

"Dad!" I gave him the dirtiest look I could. "I can't!"

"Should you take her to the emergency room?" Veronica asked from the hallway.

My dad looked down at me, "Do you think we need to go the emergency room?"

"I c-can't move!" Getting up and walking to the car was out of the question for me.

My mom left the room and my dad gave me an ultimatum. He told me, "If you slow down your breathing, then we don't have to go the emergency room – but if you don't, we are going."

"Dad! I can't!" *I would if I could, trust me.*

My mom came back with a wet washcloth that I threw over my face. I felt the droplets seep into my pores, mixing in with all my tears.

"Georgia, if you keep hyperventilating, you'll pass out," my dad said. *WHAT?!*

That statement made me do the opposite of what he wanted; I started breathing harder and faster. The thought of passing out only made me panic even more. I felt like I wasn't getting any oxygen at all, even when I took the wet washcloth off my face. I had the worst headache of my life, and everything was just getting worse.

"Okay Georgia," my dad said, picking me up. "We're going to the emergency room. Let's go."

"Should I come, too?" my mom asked, following us into the living room.

"No, you stay with Veronica," my dad insisted.

"Okay, honey, I love you and everything is going to be okay," she said hugging me, but I could sense the emptiness in those words. Even she wasn't completely sure of them.

My dad grabbed a pair of shoes and a sweatshirt for me as we rushed out of the house. I was still hyperventilating by the time we got to the car, but during the ride I started to calm down. I don't know if it was the cool night wind in my face or listening to cars zooming past each other. Whatever it was, it worked.

When we pulled into the UCLA hospital parking lot, my breathing was for the most part back to normal. My hands were still cramping and my heart was still beating faster than usual.

I sat in the waiting room while my dad went to the reception desk. I quickly realized that I didn't have anything. *I left my phone and chapstick at home!* What am I going to do? *Just sit here?*

I need Billy, I need my song.

"They know you're here," my dad said, sitting down in the seat across from me. In a couple of minutes he filled out the papers on the clipboard and took them back to the lady behind the desk.

"Thank you, Mr. Huston," the lady smiled at him. "We will be with your daughter as soon as possible."

That night would be the straw that broke the camel's back for me. That was the night that opened my eyes wider than they had ever been. There was a clock above the receptionist's desk that became my biggest enemy. This whole experience showed me that time is one of the most precious things to have. Once time is lost, there is absolutely no way to get it back. If you lose your phone, you call it; if you lose your iPod, you get a new one. When you lose time, there is nothing you can do.

Eight-sixteen p.m.

"Did you bring my phone or chapstick?" I asked my dad.

"I forgot," he said.

My eyes started to water again, like a toddler having a tantrum when something goes wrong. I put my head in my hands and cried. I'm so stupid; *how could I forget those?* The smallest things were throwing me off these days. But, before I knew it I was humming "Vienna."

Too bad but it's the life you lead
You're so ahead of yourself that you forgot what you need
Though you can see when you're wrong, you know
You can't always see when you're right.

Too bad, but it's the life you lead... yeah, too fricken bad. This isn't my life. I don't recognize this life at all. I don't think I'm ahead of myself, I think I'm way behind. I did forget what I need, but that's just because I am stupid and nothing goes right in my life. I would be able to see when I was right, if that were the case; I don't see it because it is simply not there. I am always wrong.

Nine-oh-two p.m.
Where did all that time go? Shouldn't I be seeing a doctor by now?

"Dad, how much longer?" I whined.
"Georgia," he said not looking up from his magazine, "they'll call us when it's our turn."
How could he just sit there and be this calm?
I soon learned how he could just sit there and be that calm. I learned that night actually. I learned that a doctor's time is much more important than anybody else's time, or at least they think that. I learned that doctors don't wait on you, you wait on them – you wait on them all night.

My bitterness towards doctors doesn't blind me. I understand that doctors have busy and hard days filled with whining patients, I really do; but I also think I have the right to be sour towards them. They aren't bad people and they don't necessarily do it on purpose, but that is simply the way it is. In most cases the patients don't come first and don't really matter on a personal level. To doctors, patients are just another illness that needs a cure, not a person who needs help. Doctors will very rarely go out of their way to help someone because, well, to put it simply, their time is more important; *remember?*

Ten-twelve p.m.
"Georgia Huston?" *Finally!*
We followed the nurse into a small room where she took my temperature, blood pressure, weight, and height. She asked me a few questions. *Does this mean I get to see a doctor now?*
"Okay, thank you Miss. If you'll have a seat in the waiting room, we will be with you as soon as possible."
My heart dropped; *no, that's not okay.* "How long will that be?" I was not going back out there without a definite answer; I have been told that "as soon as possible" shit for way too long.
"I don't know Miss, but I promise you we will be with you as soon as possible," she said, not looking up from her computer. She obviously

didn't know how stubborn I was and that I was not leaving without an answer.

I started to get an attitude, "Listen, we have been here for almost three hours. I need to see a doctor. This is getting ridiculous."

That got her attention. "Do you see how many people are in that waiting room?" she pointed, getting an attitude of her own.

"Yeah, I do actually."

"Well what makes you think you deserve special treatment? I think you should go in there and wait your turn."

"I have been waiting my turn and guess what? I am not asking for special treatment. I understand there are other people waiting. Get them to doctors, too! There are people in there who have been here since I got here, and God only knows how long they were waiting before me. Do you know who's out there waiting? There's a little baby who keeps coughing and his mother has the most devastated expression on her face that I have ever seen. There is a young girl out there who is breathing so heavily, she needs a doctor, too! We all need doctors and it's your job to get us to see one, not have us sit around here in agony, waiting for hours."

That did nothing. She didn't care; as long as she could still text her friends and drink her Starbucks. *Who cares about us?*

After another forty-five minutes they finally called me in – not that lady, another one. They brought me through the winding corridors to a random bed pushed to the side of the hallway.

That is by far one of the most depressing things to do, walk through a hospital hallway. Even if you try not to look through the open doors into rooms, you always end up seeing things you don't want to see. I have learned through my own experiences that there is nothing worse than seeing people in a hospital bed. I can look at their bandages and the IVs going into their arms and neck, and feel bad for them because that seems horrible enough. What most people might not think about is how they are feeling. I'm not talking about the physical pain of their stitches or broken hips healing; I'm talking about the emotional torment of being in a hospital bed – stuck.

If someone has never been in one, they cannot even imagine. They cannot imagine the embarrassment of having to use a bed pan or the bother of having to wait with dozens of other patients, all for the same doctor who is only there for a couple of hours during the day. They cannot imagine the letdown of pressing the button for the nurses when you really need them, and then waiting for another half hour until they actually get there, annoyed that you're bothering them. They cannot imagine being so excited when the sun comes up, opening the window shade, and realizing your only view is of a parking lot. They cannot imagine the absolute heartache of being so vulnerable, while the people you love and respect just stand by, watching sympathetically and helplessly. They cannot imagine.

I lay down in my bed on wheels in the middle of the hallway and closed my eyes. I put my sweater over my face and just listened. I heard heels clacking, creaky carts being wheeled, and people with walkers scooting by me. *Hospitals suck.*
Ten-fifty-two p.m.

Doctor Ten didn't know anything, no surprise there. He felt my back and "took a look" at my films, but he couldn't have put that much attention into them. I knew that from the fact that he spent as little time with us as my dad would let him get away with. So, as a result of the few minutes he spent with us, he barely looked at my X-rays or MRIs, so who knows if he might have seen something had he given them all of his attention.

That was always a big thing, the "what if." *What if you looked at it in a different light? What if you had your morning coffee instead of that smoothie?* The most discouraging thing about this doctor, who I honestly don't know the name of, that's how influential he was in my life, was how bored he seemed while we explained my symptoms. All he told us was that I'd had a panic attack. *Oh really?*

We knew I had a panic attack. That was pretty obvious. We just didn't know why – just like we knew I was going through a lot of pain, we just didn't know why.

He didn't refer us to anyone; he didn't give us a printout of information on panic attacks, nothing. There was no determination in his eyes while he "took a look" at my films, no regret in his eyes as he told us he didn't see anything abnormal, and no hope in his eyes as he watched me get up from my bed on wheels and limp away. I was just a patient to him. I was another problem, not a person.

When we went home it was just becoming light outside, our first of many slumber parties at the ER.

Mom was waiting up in the armchair right next to the door; *big surprise.*

"How'd it go, honey?" she asked, standing up and walking towards me, I'm guessing for a hug, but I walked coldly past her.

"Horrible."

I didn't have to go to school that day. I was missing a lot of school lately.

That was the day that my dad came in and told me that I had unlimited texting. I had a cell phone, but I had never been allowed to text on it, which is what everyone did. I couldn't figure out for the life of me why he suddenly let me text, without my asking or anything, but I didn't question it. That was the last thing I was going to do – I just went with it.

I looked through my address book and put a check next to each name that I wanted to share this news with, and sent a mass and excited text out to everyone. I was the only one in my group of friends not allowed to text, and probably the only one in the whole school for that matter. Everyone was just as happy as I was that I could now.

I eventually figured out my dad's reasoning. My friend's mom told me about a year later. As much as he was against texting, and still is, he knew it was the only practical way to stay in touch with my friends. I was missing so much and not spending as much time with friends as I should be, but he still wanted me in the loop and talking to people; so he gave me unlimited texting. He is the most difficult man ever sometimes, but he has always wanted me to live every experience to the fullest. He has always made such an effort to have me do everything possible, and my teenage years' experiences were no exception.

There was a soccer scrimmage that evening, so I had to get up for that.

"Where were you today?" Tracy asked when I showed up during stretching. I was in my uniform and shorts, but no cleats or shin guards. Just my school Vans.

"I wasn't feeling well."

I left it at that. It didn't make any sense to go into the details of why I really wasn't there. They already knew I had the pars defect. Explaining my night in the hospital would just be a pain. I always did that, always kept it secret, and never really let outsiders see my true life.

"Oh! You missed it! Mr. Taylor brought pictures today of him in high school," Cathrine informed me.

"Why is it taking you guys so long to stretch? Let's go ladies!" Our coach came up behind us. "Georgia, can you get the balls together for us?"

That's all I ended up being for the team, the water girl and the girl who chased the balls after wild kicks. That's why I did those nine weeks of conditioning and came to every practice without fail. *That's exactly why.*

As I started to walk around the field getting our stranded balls, the pain shot down my leg and I almost fell over it was so bad. It came out of nowhere in mid-step. But I kept going. *If they knew I could barely even walk around, how in the world would they think I was ready to play next season?* I held back tears and bit my lip as I carried on; *I refuse to let anyone see me as weak.*

There were a couple of balls over where the boys' soccer team was practicing; *great.* I pulled my phone out of my pocket to look like I was texting while I walked by them all stretching in a circle. I thought I could just sneak by, but Mr. Taylor, my English teacher, was the coach.

"Hey Georgia! Where were you today?" he shouted, even though I wasn't that far away. He had a way of embarrassing people on purpose, but everyone still loved him.

"I was sick," I said, putting my phone back in my pocket. *My cover's blown.*

"Was it your back again?" he asked sympathetically. *How'd he know?! Did my dad send another e-mail to all my teachers without telling me? Not cool.*

"Yeah, but I'm fine," and I tried to end it there. I put my head down and kept walking. The thing I hated most during all of that was the extra attention I got.

"Are you gonna be at school tomorrow?" Darren asked me. *Great, now I have the attention of the whole team.*

"Yeah, I will."

That was one thing that was for sure at Notre Dame. There was no way you could slip in and out of that campus. People are there twenty-four/seven and they all want to know your business. The more people who asked what was up with me, the shorter and simpler my story got.

I was not in class the next day. I had forgotten that I had to go to Paul's to get my body cast. *Fun.* I went in there blind; I had no idea what to expect, nothing.

My dad and I walked into the colorful waiting room which was always empty, and were greeted by the receptionist. She immediately sent us to our room, where we sat down and waited for my buddy, Paul. When he came in my heart stopped. Paul was lugging this big white hollow block thing. *That can't be for me.*

"Hey guys," he said, setting the block on a table in the corner and then sitting on the chair across from me.

"Hi Paul," I said, hesitantly eyeing the elephant in the room; the white hollow block in the corner. "That's not it, right?"

He looked at me, then at the white block, then back at me and shrugged his shoulders.

Before I knew it he was strapping me in. It was like a medieval torture machine from the movies, no joke. There was a front and back that were connected by Velcro straps, so it was like a shell being put around me. It started from under my breast to my belly and pelvis, same size on the back, and went down my right leg until just before my knee. There was no space in between the body cast part and the leg cast part – it just went down, forcing me to be straight as an arrow. He told me to sleep with it, take showers with it, everything. There was no excuse for it not to be on me.

He brought me over to the mirror and had me take a look. "It's really tight," I said under my breath.

"It's supposed to be, don't let it be any looser," he said while he motioned for me to look in the mirror.

The mirror – my heart sank deeper than it ever had before. My heart wasn't in my chest anymore; or in my belly or in my feet. I don't know where my heart went, but wherever it went was better than where I was at that moment.

"If you follow me, Jimmy, you can pay over here," Paul said leading my dad out of the room. I was alone with the mirror.

Where did my figure go? I had always been in shape and had an extremely small waist.

Where did I go? I didn't see myself in that mirror. I don't know who I saw, but it wasn't me. I didn't see the girl who loves to take her beautiful dogs on walks. I didn't see the girl who had every sports trophy she'd ever won proudly displayed in her room. What I definitely didn't see was a girl who was going to get any attention from boys, that was for sure.

My eyes started to water. *I look like a freak.* When I put my clothes on I looked even bulkier and even more like a rectangular block. *This cannot be happening.*

But, in the back of my mind I knew that this was in fact happening and that this was my life. To walk out of the room, since I was held rigid – even my right leg couldn't bend at the hip – I invented a sort of rocking motion to get from one place to another. If I would step with my left foot, my whole middle section would fall forward because it had to stay in line with my right leg which was behind me. Then when I would pull my right leg up to catch up with my left, my whole upper body would rock back. I felt like a cuckoo clock when the dolls come out and bend over to kiss, and their whole mid-section works together and there is no flexibility whatsoever in the way they move.

I did my rocking walk out into the waiting room and then out to the car. Getting into the car was a challenge in itself. I literally could not bend at the hip, I was a plank. So, we put the seat as far back as it could go, so it was like a flat bed, and somehow I managed to wiggle myself in there.

I lay there looking up at the ceiling of the car, the only place that I could look. I couldn't see out the window or anything. It was a silent car ride. Nothing either of us could have said would have made the situation any better.

My dad helped me into his bed, which took ten times as long as usual. When I said I was fine and he left the room, I wanted to get something to eat. That was when I realized that I was stuck. I was like a turtle or a roly-poly bug when they get turned on their back and their legs are running in the air. That's what it felt like and it was the most depressing and helpless feeling ever, just to lie there and not even be able to turn. All I could do was grab the nearest blanket and put it over my face.

That blanket wasn't enough, I needed more. I reached for every blanket, sheet, and pillow I could get to and stacked them on top of me, heaviest things on the bottom. With each layer of soft linens or knitted blankets, I felt safer and safer. As the wall between me and the rest of the world got thicker and higher, I felt more relaxed, but my mind was still wandering in the dark and quiet space I had created for myself.

> *Slow down, you crazy child and take the phone off the*
> *hook*
> *and disappear for a while.*
> *It's alright, you can afford to lose a day or two*
> *When will you realize, Vienna waits for you?*

The fact is that I don't really have a choice whether I slow down or not. I am past the point of slowing down, I am stopped. Everything I have has been taken off the "hook" because of all this; everything. Disappear for a while... disappear. That's all I can do at this point, disappear. I feel like I can't afford to lose a day or two because every day or two that pass I get more and more depressed and lost. I get more confused and uncomfortable in my own body with every tick of the clock. Vienna might be waiting for me, but it's going to have to wait for a while more because I can't even get out of this bed.

That night I didn't sleep at all. I kept thinking about how school was going to be the next day. *How was I going to make it up the stairs; sit down in class?* It was the last day of our fall semester finals and I only had one exam, so it was going to be a quick day, *thank god.* Unfortunately it was in biology, my absolute worst subject ever. So, besides being stressed about taking my hardest final, in the class with my lowest grade, with my least understanding of the material – I also had to worry about how I was going to get around with this stupid body cast.

I started to cry. I was in bed alone, facing the wall in my dark room and crying my eyes out. I started to chew on my pillowcase, tears pouring down my face. I closed my eyes and imagined what Vienna looked like.

I had never seen pictures of it, but I had an interesting way of illustrating what I imagined it looked like. I thought it was like in the movie "The Sound of Music." The Von Trapp family lived in Austria. Vienna, obviously, is in Austria, so I figured that Vienna should look something like the settings in "The Sound of Music." I pictured little churches on grass hills that go for miles, small houses with stairs leading all the way down to the water of calm rivers, and the cutest little old fashioned buildings and family owned businesses ever. Turns out that the real Vienna is absolutely nothing like that, or at least isn't anymore. But that really doesn't matter. Like I said before, Vienna can be whatever I want it to be.

Chapter Eight

When I woke up I was in so much pain that I could hardly stand it. It wasn't the usual pain of my back or leg, which of course always hurt. My body ached everywhere. Sleeping in a body cast is like sleeping on the floor, but somehow the hardwood floor is rubbing against your entire body all night long. My friends and sister will definitely attest to the fact that I am a rough sleeper and I am always kicking or moving around; I also sleep talk but that's beside the point. So, with me wiggling around as best I could in that tight hard box, I managed to get bruises and sores all over my body. It was not an easy thing to sleep in.

Getting ready in the morning turned into a huge family affair that needed everyone's help; it was chaos. We got up extra early because it would take more time to get me ready. My mom helped me get dressed, my sister made my lunch, and my dad got random things together that we asked him to find, like socks or binders.

If you just saw my upper body, you might not notice anything; it just looked like I was a little chubbier than I really was. But, my skirt showed about eight inches of my cast, which I was not happy about at all; *at least people will see a reason I'm walking the way I am.*

I went to school early that morning to go to the office. I gave them a letter from my dad explaining what was going on, or at least what we thought was going on. They were very nice and accommodating. They gave me an elevator pass so that I didn't have to use the stairs, and then they gave me a note to give to my one teacher of the day.

When I found the classroom that was assigned for my biology final, I went in and found my group of friends from that class. Marisa immediately ran up to me, "Oh my gosh! What happened?!" She grabbed my backpack and led me to my seat.

Cody said – louder than he had to – "What the hell happened to you?"

I wobbled over to where they were sitting. "This is the body cast I was telling you about."

"How are you going to sit down?" Braden asked me, pulling the chair out for me. I had no idea how I was going to sit down, and now that more and more people were huddling around my desk, I started to get more and more nervous. Being the klutz that I am, I just knew that I would end up embarrassing myself in front of everyone, and this class was half tenth graders, too.

I decided just to stand for this final. In the back of the room there were counters to do experiments on. I found one near a window and that was where I took my final; I was standing for almost two hours.

That final was difficult, but I had a solid "C" so I knew my grade wasn't going up or down significantly. I've always been a fast test taker, so I finished this test pretty early, especially since I wasn't trying that hard. I remember drawing a palm tree I could see from my window. It was a rough sketch in pen on a piece of scratch paper, but I remember being pretty happy with it.

That night I was feeling pretty down. I was looking at myself in the mirror in this stupid cast and feeling extremely depressed. I decided that since I was injured and this was indeed a cast, I should get it signed like people do when they break an arm or leg; *why not?*

I got a bunch of Sharpies and went into my dad's office. "Dad?" I asked, holding out a marker, "can you please sign my cast?" He laughed and put a "kick me" sign on my back.

I found my mom who wrote, "Feel better soon sweetie! Love, Mom."

Every signature from someone I loved and every splash of color on my solid white cast got me a little less depressed. I started carrying markers around with me and asking everyone.

The next night we had dinner plans with our close family friends, the Sitzers. My mom was best friends with Briana, so she and her husband Charlie were like my second parents. Their son had been my best friend since diapers. Jordan and I were the same age and we did absolutely everything together; we even went on family road trips with each other. He was one of those friends you would invite to something you don't even want to go to, because you know that if he's there, it'll be fun.

So, even though I wasn't feeling well, I sucked it up because I didn't want to miss a chance to see him. I put on my sweatpants and t-shirt that I used to wear to bed because those were the only things that would fit over my body cast. I put my hair up in a classic ponytail because I'd really stopped trying to look good since I got my body cast.

We went to El Rancho, which is where we always went. It's a friendly little neighborhood Mexican restaurant that Jordan and I grew up in. They were already sitting in our usual big round corner booth – they always got there before us.

"Hey guys!" Charlie called out, getting up to hug us.

"Is a pars defect permanent?" Briana asked curiously.

"Well it can be if it's not treated," my dad answered. "But, we're trying to avoid that with this body cast."

The waiter brought me lemonade with no ice, "Here you go, Georgia." I always loved the way he said my name. All the people who worked there knew us and our usual orders, and we knew all of them.

"*Gracias* Tally," I smiled.

"How long do you have to wear it?" Jordan asked. We were in our own little private corner.

"We don't know yet," I shrugged, trying to pretend it didn't bother me when it really did.

"Can you still swim?"

"It's waterproof, but I don't know if I can really swim," I said thinking about it.

"Is it hard to get around?" he asked, feeling the part of my cast that was on my leg. A lot of people wanted to feel what it was made of.

"Very, it's so embarrassing," I said with a light laugh.

"Don't be embarrassed," he said looking at me. "You gotta do what you gotta do."

That made me blush for some reason, so I changed the subject. "Did you check for the penny yet?"

He laughed. "No, I was waiting for you."

Since we went there almost once a week for the past twelve years, we had an ongoing game where we would hide a penny in the most unsuspecting places and then on the next visit we would see if it was still there. Sometimes it was, sometimes it wasn't. For some reason we got a little sad whenever it wasn't there, but our parents would always give us a new penny and we'd figure out a new hiding spot.

"Where should we put this one? How about behind the water cooler?" Jordan asked.

He started to stand on the seat, but I pulled him back down.

"No," I whispered looking at George, the owner, behind the counter. "Don't let George see you."

When the penny was successfully put in place and we were ready to go, I asked Jordan to sign my cast. "Yeah, sure."

He was really into graffiti then, so on the back of my cast he did his graffiti signature; a signature that would get a lot of questions from the kids at my private Catholic school.

Among our closest family friends were the Bagdadis. My parents had been friends with them since before I was born so I never had a life without the Bagdadis; *thank god.* Phyllis and Henri were the grandparents, but they are not what you would expect grandparents to be. They are in shape, energetic, amazingly kind people. Their beautiful daughter Jojo married the most charming man ever, Russell (my sister and I were the flower girls at their wedding). Together Jojo and Russ had the talented and soon to be famous Sean, who was four at the time of all this.

This particular family really made me laugh and be happy when no one else could. They had a gorgeous weekend beach house right on the shore of Oxnard. Their backyard was the ocean. It was two stories and just beautiful, and was where I spent many weekends during all of this. They could tell I needed to get my mind off things and have a little vacation, so Jojo and Sean would pick me up on Friday nights or Saturday mornings and we would make the ninety minute car ride to Oxnard. Phyllis and Henri were usually there already and Russ would come up when he could get off work.

That beach house became my sanctuary. Even thinking about that place relaxes me. As soon as we would exit the freeway we were automatically welcomed by the cool breeze and beautiful houses on the water. Everything was always so nice there.

The weekend after finals is always the best; we get three and a half days off, and there is absolutely no pressure about school. So, the evening after finals, Jojo and Sean were in my driveway and ready to go. But this would be my first long car ride in my body cast.

We put my bags in the trunk and moved the front seat back so I could lie down. Sean was in a car seat in the middle, so my head was right where his feet were. While we were driving I couldn't look up at the strawberry fields we passed or the marinas full of boats. I could just close my eyes and picture the scenery that I had grown so familiar with.

Sean had dozens of sing-a-long CDs that Jojo would play for him over and over again. Jojo's a silly lady, so after a while she and I memorized the words and we would belt out these absolutely ridiculous songs. They had names like "I Need a Nap" and "Bad Broccoli."

Jojo became one of my best friends. I would also play her some of my music and show her pictures of cute celebrity boys. She thought most of the same boys were cute, but we had extremely different taste in music and she would make that clear. She would tell me how my artists "copied" her artists' styles and songs. I would just roll my eyes even after hearing the songs and realizing how similar they were.

That car ride was long and hard; each hour that goes by in a body cast feels like three. I would toss and turn but couldn't get comfortable. I am naturally a very fidgety person and being strapped down in a cast drove me crazy. The pain was killing me, but I wasn't about to complain.

When we got to their house I had to wait for Jojo to come around and help me out; I hated being helpless. Phyllis was in her usual spot on a chair in their little gated yard.

"Hey guys!" she waved. I couldn't see her face under her sun hat, but she had a voice that you could just tell had a huge smile behind it.

"Ammie!" Sean cried as he ran through the gate and into her arms.

I offered to help Jojo with some of the bags, but she gave me a look so I followed Sean. A small white yappy dog came running and started barking at my feet. "Hey Potter," I started to bend down to pet him but my cast wouldn't let me. I looked around to see if anyone saw and was thankful that no one had except for their black Sharpe, Harley.

"Hi Miss Georgia, how are you?" Phyllis asked embracing me.

"I've been better," I answered hugging her back. "Where's Henri?"

"Where do you think?" She smiled. *Napping.*

That was a great day, but so were most of my days at the beach house. Everyone there signed my cast, even Sean. Russell drew the coolest design on it, one that he made up. He called it a "zoom" and it was like a collage of designs that all fit in a really cool way. I became the only other person to master a "zoom" and Russell and I still proudly send our "zooms" to each other.

That night Jojo and I went to Blockbuster. She always let me pick out movies to watch together. I introduced her to so many new cute romantic comedies that she completely fell in love with. She loved all of them except for one that was an absolute disaster.

In the morning we walked to this tiny breakfast place in our PJs, just Sean, Jojo, and me. We were usually the only ones there in PJs and we always had to wait a while for a table because it was packed. I would get blueberry pancakes that were not that great, but it was the idea of going there with them that always got me excited.

Chapter Nine

My first day of the new semester; new classes, new teachers, everything. Only one of my classes had seen me in my body cast, so it was still relatively new to everyone else. I was thankful that Solene and I had the same first period, so I had a buddy for my first class; Ms. Loya, Sacraments.

I'd had Ms. Loya the previous semester for religion so I didn't even think to check what room she was in. I just assumed that it would be the same classroom. So, when the bell rang I led Solene to my religion building. Using the stairs took a long time but I knew Ms. Loya wouldn't mind if I was late. Going up stairs I would keep my right leg hanging straight down – like I had a choice – and march up with my left leg. I had an elevator pass from the dean, but it was all the way on the other side of the building and would take even longer. I just worked my way up one step at a time while patient Solene waited at the top of the stairs with my backpack.

"This is it," I motioned to room fifty-two. She opened the door for me so I smiled and waddled through – right into a class full of seniors. Both of our faces got red as we looked around completely confused. Without saying a word we both backed out and started laughing. We were completely embarrassed but it was funny, too.

"I don't think that's her room," Solene said as the tardy bell rang. *Great, late on the first day of class.*

"I'm so sorry," I said, checking my schedule. It turned out she'd changed classrooms and I'd just never checked.

After asking a senior and feeling extremely stupid, we found where our new room was. We walked in during morning announcements on the PA system and I will never forget the reaction of those in the room. Ms. Loya ran over and made the biggest fuss over me. Apparently my dad had e-mailed all my teachers telling them what happened and that I would be in a body cast; *great*.

But since they all knew ahead of time, at least I didn't have to explain it to them in front of the whole class right? – Wrong.

"Oh my God, Georgia! I am so sorry!" Ms. Loya said standing extremely close to me. "Your dad e-mailed me. How are you feeling?"

"I'm fine," I said blushing, as I looked around at all of the new and intimidating faces. "I'm sorry we're late...." But before I could explain that we'd gotten lost she interrupted.

"Oh, it's completely fine; you take all the time you need getting to my class." Since she'd assumed we were late because of my body cast, we just went with it. "And thank you for helping Georgia out. Do you need a note for your teacher?"

"No, I'm in this class, too."

"Oh! That's perfect. Where do you want to sit?"

I looked around the room and pointed to the only open back corner. "Can we sit there?"

"Yes of course," she said leading us to our corner. "Can you sit in the desk?" She eyed the bottom of my cast sticking out from under my skirt.

"I can try," I said, still checking out the rest of the curious new faces; *ahh yes, my favorite thing in the world – extra attention.*

I tried to wiggle my way into the seat of the small one-piece metal desk from as many angles and directions as we could think of. Finally Ms. Loya offered to pull her chair up to the desk for me to use instead of the built-in chair.

Since I couldn't bend at the waist there was no way for me to actually sit down. I invented, with the help of some of my classmates, a unique way of resting on a seat. I would come at the chair from the right side and bend my left leg and sit on the chair with my left butt cheek. Then with my right leg, I would put my knee on the ground in a sort of kneeling fashion. It was not very comfortable at all and extremely difficult to balance on, but it was the most normal looking way to blend into a classroom – that's all I really wanted to do, just blend in.

All day, question after question; and they were all the same questions over and over again, which made it extremely frustrating. Also, since I was in new classes that day with new people, I didn't have friends in all of my classes yet. In those I had to carry my own backpack, step up and talk to the new teacher, and limp/waddle around the room for myself. People were very nice, interested, and helpful, but one of my biggest flaws is that I usually don't ask or accept help when I need it, so I was on my own.

Soccer practice felt like it was never going to end because even though I was in a body cast, I still volunteered to collect all the stray balls. The nights were getting cold as winter grew closer and all the team would donate their sweatshirts and beanies to me. They gave me a pair of gloves, too, and then I was on my own. I could see my breath as it left my lips and I could feel all of my muscles tightening in the breeze, but I still wanted to be out there.

I could tell how much they appreciated having me there. They would all tell me repeatedly I was part of the team. I went to the sleepovers, the dinners, and was on all the bus rides. I never felt left out because I was always on the field with them, even if I wasn't playing.

Slow down, you're doing fine,
You can't be everything you want to be before your time
Although it's so romantic on the borderline tonight
Tonight....

I'm going as slow as I possibly can, I can't go any faster. My mobility is so limited and I'm always at the mercy of this stupid cast. If I was doing fine, wouldn't that mean I would be a little happier? Fine means acceptable, satisfactory, etc.; I don't fit any of the synonyms for "fine." I'm not trying to do anything before my time; I'm not trying to skip anything. I was never someone to go above and beyond on anything; I always did the bare minimum in schoolwork, housework, etc. I am the last person who would try to be anything before my time. I just want to enjoy my life like everyone else my age.

I want to worry about someone telling my crush that I like him, where to get the cheapest movie tickets, and which mall we should go to on the weekends – Topanga or Fashion Square? I am fourteen, I shouldn't be worrying about whether I'm going to be able to get out of bed in the morning; but I am. To me, the word romantic means idealistic and borderline means unclear. They are both so vague to me right now, they are open-ended. Open ended, just like my fractured spine and body cast. Open ended – yeah, open-ended sucks.

"Come on, Georgia," my dad said turning on the lights in my room. The light burned through my closed eyelids and I moaned, stretching out my arms over my head. "Jenny's here." *Jenny?*

I walked out wiping my eyes and sure enough, my friend Jenny was sitting in the living room.

"What are you doing here?" I asked sleepily.

"Your dad told me to come over," she replied, looking at my dad.

"I thought you'd want to go see the new Jonas Brothers movie," he said smiling. He looked so excited to see my reaction.

I didn't want to see it – well actually I wanted to see it, but I didn't want to go out and see it. Leaving the house had become a huge ordeal thanks to the body cast, but so did everything I guess. Even getting up to go to the bathroom was a huge hassle. I hated going out of the house. I got enough stares and questions at school, *why would I go out of my way for more?*

Looking at my dad's face and how excited he was, I couldn't say no. He looked so pleased that he'd thought of a way to make me happy, so I just smiled and said yes.

I put on a sleeping t-shirt and soccer sweatpants, my usual attire, and put my hair up in a bun. I didn't wear my hair down at all while I was in my body cast; *since I feel ugly I must look ugly, too.* I had Jenny put my Uggs on for me, because I couldn't even bend over to put on my own socks and shoes. I was helpless.

My sister came, too, so it was my dad, Veronica, Jenny, and me. I wasn't thrilled about going with my little sister or dad, but it didn't really matter when I was in the body cast, because I would be embarrassed all of the time anyway.

We went to the Galleria Arclight, so it was a really nice theater. The movie was just a recording of their concerts, but in 3D, so we got those cool glasses.

Whenever I can, I always sit in the very last row of movie theatres; I don't know why, I just hate people being able to see what I'm doing when I can't see them. I know they wouldn't be watching me, they would be watching the movie, but I just don't like the feeling.

I laid down in a very odd fashion. I was half on the floor and half on the chair, and we waited for the movie to start. When it did start, Jenny and I looked at each other in awe; she liked them even more than I did.

These boys were so athletic, cute, and talented; even my dad was impressed. They were such great entertainers and they were doing gymnastics and flips on stage. The whole time Jenny and I were singing every lyric to every song, we felt so cool. We didn't care who else was in the theatre.

I will never forget that hour and a half. That was the hour and a half when I was myself again. When the lights went out in the theatre and I disappeared into the darkness, so did my body cast. I was not "the girl with the broken back" anymore. In that hour and a half, I was Georgia Huston, lost in the fantasy world of handsome guys flexing their muscles and singing happy songs about love.

When the credits came on the screen and the lights came up I felt lost. As I saw the faces of those around me, I shot back into reality. I could feel my right knee getting sore from kneeling on the cold floor, and my body ached from rubbing against the cast.

My number one model was my mom. She was the one who I had the most drawings of. No matter what she was doing or what mood she was in, when I would ask if I could draw her, the answer was always yes.

She was working on her computer when I asked this time and she said she was busy, but if I wanted to draw her like that, she would stay still for me.

I sat across from mom and her laptop at the dining room table. I put down my pad of notebook paper and picked up my pencil. I took one hard look at her, taking my time to notice every crevice and freckle. She would look up awkwardly while I stared at her.

When I am drawing people, the very first thing I draw are the eyes. I think that the eyes are the foundation of every face. The first place someone looks when they meet someone is into their eyes. When you want to know how someone is feeling, you look into their eyes. Everyone says that eyes are the window to the soul, and I agree with that. You can tell everything about how someone's feeling through looking into their eyes.

To make a person look right, you have to completely capture their eyes; the shape, the wrinkles, the lashes. Through the eyes you can capture the innocence of a baby or the stress of someone middle-aged. The eyes are what shows when someone is sad, or when someone is laughing. The mouth and cheeks help, but it's mostly in the eyes.

I focused on the curve of her pupils as they focused on the small print of the computer screen. I drew each eyelash in its own direction and length. I illustrated how deep her eyelids were with a dark shadow. I made her eyebrows as thin and distinct as they really were and I added a few lines to define her face. I put a few wrinkles under her eyes because she was squinting and I made her hair as big and wild as it really was.

I rubbed my dry finger over the dark areas of her face, and then did it with another finger, softer in the light spots. Shading gave her face depth so it didn't just look like an outlined cartoon. I never showed her that drawing, I don't even know where it is now. All I know is that I did it, and I was embarrassed by it.

"Hey there, Miss Georgia," Jojo said grinning ear to ear as she opened the door into my parents' room. I was lying on the bed like a zombie staring up at the ceiling in darkness, the only light being the television that I wasn't watching.

"Hi Jojo," I said, not smiling but giving a kind look. "What are you doing here?"

"I want to spend time with you guys!" she said sitting on the bed. "I wanted to see you, Georgia."

"I'm not much to see right now," I whined, looking away from her.

"Come on," she sighed, hitting the bed with her hand. "We are all going to dinner and I would love for you to join us."

Before I knew it I was sitting in the dimly lit, crowded, and noisy *Las Fuentes* in Reseda. This restaurant is always packed and they don't seat you, which means you have to find your own table. The thing to do is send one person to place your order and then everyone else spreads out around the restaurant and keeps their eyes open for people leaving. But, it's not that easy, because everyone else there wants that table just as badly as you. It's always a jungle at *Las Fuentes,* but it's worth it.

The inside of this place is so funky and artsy. The colors are all bright and there are big fruit sculptures hanging from the ceiling. There are different tropical birds carved into the backs of the chairs. Everything about this place is fun but chaotic – the perfect place to trigger a panic attack....

"So how's school going?" Jojo asked, sitting down across from me.

"I wouldn't know," I said semi-rudely sipping my lime *Jarritos* drink.

"How much have you been missing?"

"I didn't go all last week."

"Wow," Jojo said sitting back in her chair, "are you keeping up?"

"As best she can," my dad answered for me.

"How are your grades?"

"I don't know," I lied. My school posts all of our grades online, so literally when the teacher grades a test and inputs it to the computer, my online grade updates simultaneously. I had been looking at my grades almost every day and watching them go downhill, but whenever anyone asked about my grades I'd just play dumb and say that I wasn't sure.

"We've got to give credit to the teachers," my dad said. "They are doing everything they can and have been very understanding in this whole situation – and for that matter the whole school has." *That's what you think, dad. Yes, they are being nice, but you don't feel the eyes glued to my back and hear the whispers, the rumors.*

"I'm sure you'll get right back into the swing of things soon," Jojo said hopefully.

"Setenta y cinco. Seventy-five. *Setenta y cinco."*

"That's us," my dad said standing up. "Veronica can you come help me, please?"

When they left to get our food my mom tried to change the conversation. "How's Sean?"

"Oh he's great," Jojo smiled, "he's going to a sports camp by the beach house every Sunday."

"That's great. How's he liking it?"

"He loves it," she said.

"Why didn't he come tonight?" I asked.

"Because you know if he came that it would be all about him. I wanted tonight to be all about you, Miss Georgia."

"I love Sean. He can come whenever he wants."

"I know, Georgia."

Halfway through the meal I started to feel a lot more sweat on my forehead. I thought it might just be because I was sitting/squatting for longer than usual and it was pretty hot in *Las Fuentes*. I started to notice some spots in my vision and everything got darker all of a sudden. It was as if I could feel the mood change in my body and outside it, at the exact same time. The constant murmur of voices started to get louder, but less clear as I dropped my fork and put my face into my hands.

I could feel a numbness starting to inhabit my body. It started in my right hand and I felt it slowly move up and spread into my face and jaw. I was no longer part of the table's conversation; I was in my own conversation. It was an argument of power and control between my body and the intruder that I have become all too familiar with.

I started out strong; *no this is not going to happen right now – not in front of Jojo.*

"Georgia, are you okay?" Veronica asked, causing all the heads at the table to turn.

I looked up and nodded.

When I put my head back down, my strong voice and sense of authority slowly weakened; *okay, just hide it – you can hide it, Georgia.*

My mom reached into my lap and squeezed my leg. I faked a reassuring smile; the conversation continued as I secretly wiped my tears and hid my sniffling nose.

Then all of a sudden, like a flash flood breaking through a dam, I was overwhelmed with a sense of confusion, anxiety, and terror. I bit down on my hand as a cry of fear tried to escape from my body.

"Peaches, what's wrong?!" my mom asked, alarmed.

All I did was close my eyes while I sobbed.

"Georgia?" my dad said, standing up and coming over to me.

Veronica put her hand on my shoulder sympathetically and all I could do was shake my head until she took it off.

"Georgia," my dad said sternly. "You have to talk to us. You have to tell us what's going on."

I opened my mouth to speak but nothing came out. My vocal cords were not working. I shook my head again.

"Yes, Georgia," he said calmly. "You have to."

"I'm having a panic attack," I whispered with closed eyes. Saying it out loud only seemed to give it more power.

"What?" they all asked at the same time, all leaning in so they could hear me repeat it.

I took a deep breath and tried again. "I'm having a panic attack," I said, probably even less clearly than before.

"What?" my dad asked.

"She's having a panic attack," Veronica translated.

"Oh my gosh! Honey," my mom cried out sympathetically as she grabbed my hand again. "What do we do?" she asked, looking up at my dad.

He immediately said, "Veronica, you get all this food and put it in to-go containers, quickly! I'm gonna bring the car around front. Lynn and Jojo, bring Georgia out and wait for me."

The ride back was a blur. The trip from *Las Fuentes* to my house is about twenty minutes with L.A. traffic. I was sitting between my mom and Jojo, who were both holding my hands and stroking my hair, face, anything they could reach. Everyone was talking to me and telling me to calm down, but it was impossible to understand exactly what they were saying over my fast paced breath and heartbeat.

During panic attacks I was the only one I was worried about; I was the only one I could worry about. I had never been afraid of my body, I had always been confident and comfortable, but now I had no idea what my body was capable of. *If I can't control myself, then who can?*

Everybody just shut up and stop talking to me. There's nothing any of you can do to help; there's not even anything that I can do.

When we got home I immediately went into my parents' room as fast as I could, but I was in a body cast, so that doesn't say much. The cool silk sheets comforted my left cheek as I sank into the bed in the darkness. *What's out there? What is behind the darkness?*

I always wondered what I was not seeing behind the darkness; *what am I missing?* Darkness is a strange thing. Darkness can look like it is never ending and go for miles, when there could really be a wall two inches from your face. *How would you know?*

I was in the dark, not just in my parents' room with the lights off, but I was in the dark period. *Were my health questions going to be answered miles away or in two inches?* I wouldn't know, I was in the dark so everything looked the same.

In a blink it seemed like the room was filled with pairs of eyes just staring at me. My mom was trying to soothe me by stroking my hair and Jojo was gently rubbing my back.

"I need ice," I yelled into the bed through my chattering teeth.

"What?" my dad barked at me.

Ah! Why doesn't anyone ever understand me?!

That was such a frustrating thing for me, being the only one who could really access my mind. The fact that I couldn't communicate with anyone was heartbreaking. The last thing I wanted to do was repeat myself, but I had to.

"Ice," I whispered again.

"What?"

"She said, 'ice,'" Veronica repeated to my dad.

I thought the ice might help. I thought it could bring my focus to something else and distract me. I put the ice on my forehead and waited for it to melt down my face and into my pores. I wanted it to pour into my eye sockets and through the crease in my lips, but I couldn't wait. My patience was just not there, and never really was during panic attacks. I threw the ice off and started making screeching noises.

"Georgia, what's going on?" Jojo asked me calmly. I was just moaning over and over again, trying to tune out the chaos in my mind. *How could my mind be so blank, but so busy at the same time?*

The shooting pain went down my right leg and I screamed. I tried to grab my leg, but I couldn't reach it because of my body cast. I tried to turn over in the bed, but I couldn't because of my body cast. I felt an itch on my back, but I couldn't scratch it because of my body cast.

I am so beyond over this. I reached over to the side of my body cast and pulled off the first two Velcro straps.

"Georgia, what are you doing?!" my dad caught my hand and pulled it away from my only way to freedom. Not being able to pull it off made my body ache that much more. I was feeling claustrophobic and trapped. I had to get out.

I pulled my arm away from my dad and with my eyes still closed I started scratching at the straps. I didn't start at the top – my eyes were closed so I started in the middle – so I was still trapped. My eyes were always closed during panic attacks, always.

"Georgia, you can't do that," my dad said.

"I ha-a-a-v-e t-o-o-o," I said, my voice shaking just as much as my body was.

"You can't...."

"I have to!" I screamed at him and then as soon as those words escaped my mouth I started sobbing as loudly as I ever have.

After that I could feel the hesitant hands slowly unstrapping me. When they pulled the top shell off of me I felt so relieved that I immediately rolled off the bottom shell and onto the bed.

That was the first time in a while that my body felt comfortable. That was the first time I sank into a bed and could feel the sheets wrapping all the way around me. *Was this a bed or a cloud?* Anything would be a cloud compared to that rock hard shell.

"Georgia, here," Jojo said walking into the room. *When did she leave?* She picked up my hand and put something in it. She wrapped my fingers around a long thin cylindrical object that I immediately felt security in. I could feel the softness in it, but also the rough edged tip. I could smell the chalky scent and hear how my nail scratched the hard surface. *But, what am I supposed to do with this?*

She put this object and my hand onto a cool, smooth, flat surface that I was all too familiar with. I softly stroked it up and down, but unfortunately my body wasn't agreeing.

"Georgia, draw," Jojo said, dragging my pencil around the paper. *No, I can't draw. What the hell am I supposed to draw with my eyes closed and with my mind closed off?*

"Draw," she said again, making exaggerated motions with my hand. I viciously shook my head no. "Yes, Georgia." She sat me up and put the notebook pad in my lap, pencil in hand.

I honestly just wanted to get her off my back so I started drawing, the pain in my back intensifying with each stroke. Between my squinting eyes, the teardrops, and the darkness, I could barely even see what I was drawing. My jaw was clenched so tightly that my teeth were aching as badly as my back.

I took that charcoal pencil and did things that I had never done before. My art was always very reserved and safe. I always did what I thought would look good, not necessarily what I wanted to do. This was my first time breaking down all of my boundaries with art and just doing what I wanted to do.

Since I couldn't really see what I was drawing, that made it even easier; I just went with what I was feeling. I did take a few peeks to make sure I wasn't just making a glob, but for the most part it was just my emotions drawing, not my hand. I felt all the eyes in the room on my hand and when I felt like it was done, I allowed my eyes to join them.

The very first thing I thought of was one word; *scary*.

I had never used such strong and defining marks before; mine were usually soft and forgiving. I had drawn a hand squeezing the life out of a stress ball. That hand just happened to have full on black claws instead of fingernails. On the upper-right hand corner of the page, in big bold block letters I wrote one word; one single word that described everything: *pain*.

They were hollow letters; the blank whiteness was hiding behind the dark rough lines, spelling the one little word holding me back. It was a little word when you see it on paper and count the letters, but when you think about it, it is one of the biggest words I know. That one little word defined me and changed everything about me.

Pain is what made me feel ugly.
Pain is what made me feel scared.
Pain is what made me feel alone.

Whenever I look at that drawing I feel liberated, because not only did it teach me that drawing during a panic attack could calm me down, but that art could also teach me something about myself. Drawing became my way of communicating with myself through my chaotic mind.

Chapter Ten

When I woke up I was absolutely exhausted. That was always one of the worst feelings ever, waking up after a panic attack. Every muscle in your body aches like you wouldn't believe because, depending on your panic attack, every muscle in your body could have been strained for hours. I could also never remember falling asleep, which was a weird feeling. Looking back on the panic attacks, my memories of them were even more confusing than it probably even was at the time.

When I woke up after a panic attack, the only thing I ever wanted to do was to go back to sleep; but I never could. The total numbness that encompassed me after a panic attack was unexplainable and stopped me dead in my tracks.

I looked at my phone; *Monday, 9:14 a.m. – I guess I'm not going to school today either.*

For some reason, thinking about that made me start to cry again; today was going to be the pep rally. *How much more of my life am I going to be missing?*

> *Slow down, you crazy child*
> *and take the phone off the hook and disappear for a while.*
> *It's all right; you can afford to lose a day or two.*
> *When will you realize... Vienna waits for you?*

Slowing down is all I have right now. But how can I get any slower when I feel like I'm already stopped? I am at a dead end and I don't know what do to. I am crazy, I know. Even if my phone is on the hook I feel like I have disappeared. I feel like I have disappeared no matter what, I am just not here anymore; and will it be a while? How do you know, Billy, that it won't be forever? It's actually not all right – I don't want to lose a day or two. I don't want to lose anything, especially not time. Vienna... my fantasy land... When will it stop waiting? When will it find me?

"Okay Georgia," my dad said coming into the room. "It's time." I looked up and saw my prison. My heart sank as I felt the iron doors shut on my cell and he gently Velcroed me into my own personal institution, my hell.

"Hey, Georgie," Veronica said as she opened the door and came into the bedroom. I winced as she thumped her backpack on the bed.

"Hey, Nacks," I replied, not looking away from the TV.

"How are you?" she asked.

"Horrible."

"Is there anything you need?" I couldn't tell if it was a hollow question, so she could stay in the room and watch some extra TV, or if she was genuinely asking.

"A life," I answered, looking at her with tears in my eyes.

"George," she said scooting toward me. "You have a life, you have a great life."

"No I don't," I said crying. "I don't see a life."

"George, everything's going to be okay," she said hugging me. I cried into her hair, a common theme throughout this experience.

Family is a funny thing. With friends you can shop around and choose who you want to spend time with, and even then if you get sick of them you can just stop being friends. With family, especially if you are a kid, you are stuck. That's what makes family so stable and supportive, but it's what also makes it fragile. Every time my sister and I get in a fight, my dad says, "You're going to be sisters for a long time, so get used to it." If I had a dollar for every time he told us that, I would be rich.

"Why don't we just take the elevator?" Marisa asked, grabbing my arm as I swayed.

"No," I shook my head, "the class is right here. It doesn't make sense to walk around the building."

"But it doesn't make sense to fall either," Raquel said from a couple of steps below me.

"I'm almost there," I said under my breath. The hallways were empty.

"No you're not, George," Marisa said sympathetically.

"But then you'll both be late to class, this is the fastest way," I said taking another step; in that body cast stairs were almost impossible to climb.

"George, we don't care about being late," Raquel said.

"Let's go to the elevator," Marisa said, nodding and taking a step down.

"No, I'm not gonna make you guys late," I said.

"Come on," Marisa was smiling at me. "I have your backpack," she teased as she held it up while running down the stairs. We took the elevator.

"You're still having pain?" Dr. Nine asked in surprise.

I nodded and said, "Even more than before the cast."

"Is the pain in the same place?"

"Yes."

"Now just to be clear," my dad added, "it's in the two spots, not just one."

"I understand," Dr. Nine said, peering through his thick glasses into my file of papers. After a couple of minutes of measuring me and just staring at my X-rays, he finally broke the silence. "Okay," he paused. "What we are going to do is send you back to Paul, remember Paul?"

"Yeah."

"We are going to take this part of the cast off," he said pointing to my right hip, "and we are going to put a hinge there."

I could see the clouds opening, the sun coming out, and the angels singing *Hallelujah. A HINGE! That meant that I could bend, right?*

"So I can bend at the hip now?" I said, trying to hide my excitement. I could see my dad smiling, too.

"No," he said as my heart sank to the floor, "the hinge is actually going to be locked."

"Why is the hinge going to be locked? Isn't that what a hinge is for, to allow movement?"

"Well, we don't want movement. That's the point of the cast."

"Then why are we putting in a hinge?" I was confused.

"We want to lock your leg at a different angle so that it's not just straight down. It's at 180 degrees right now and we are going to put it at 160 or so. The hinge is so that we can use the cast we already have and don't have to make a new one."

"Why are we doing this?" My dad was confused, too.

"To hopefully give her leg some relief so the pain can stop."

The hinge didn't end up making anything easier; life was still just as difficult maneuvering in a body cast with a locked hinge.

The long car ride to the beach house was hard; it always was. It was Super Bowl Sunday and the Bagdadis were having a party. I had a few tears as my back cramped up, but I hid them pretty well.

We were immediately welcomed the second we opened the gate. They are one of the loudest families I know and they have even louder friends, but in my opinion the louder someone is, the more fun they are.

The house wasn't packed, but there were a lot of people in there. They were all watching the football game of course, but I'm not the biggest fan of football so I found a comfy spot by the guacamole. Veronica dislikes football even more than me, so we decided to go for a walk on the beach.

Everyone loves taking walks on the beach, including me, and since I hadn't done that since getting my body cast, it sounded really good. I was in a t-shirt and soccer shorts so I was comfortable and it was nice weather. My mom didn't seem that excited to have just the two of us walking along the beach, but she let us go.

Words cannot express the joy of having the hot sand hugging your feet after being separated for so long. I felt welcomed by the warm and comforting beach; *it's been too long.*

The house is right on the beach, but that doesn't mean it is right on the water. There is quite a walk from the beginning of the sand to the ocean, and that walk is magnified when you're hurting in a body cast. All I kept thinking about was the water, and that is what kept me going, but as the ocean got closer and closer I got more and more tired.

When I got to that ocean I felt right at home. I was out of breath but as soon as I got there I walked straight in.

California beaches are beautiful, but the water is always freezing. It feels good on your feet while the sun is warming the rest of your body, but when it gets to your knees, you really start to second guess going in. If you push past that initial shock and just go for it, it's beyond refreshing and can make a good day great.

I of course was not going to be swimming in the ocean anytime soon. I knew the cast was waterproof, but I didn't know how it would be in the water; *float or sink?* Whatever the answer would be, one thing is for sure; I would be completely at the mercy of the unforgiving ocean. There was no way I would have been able to swim or control where I was going whatsoever. My body was constricted by this body cast so much that there would be nothing I would be able to do in the water but be thrown around.

In a way, that reflected my life at the moment. I'd fallen into this whole pain thing as naïve and innocent as I could have been. My fate was not up to me, just like it wouldn't have been if I had gone swimming. Whether I floated or sank would be up to doctors, I had no way of diagnosing or writing prescriptions for myself. *So what's it gonna be, docs? Are you gonna let me sink?*

In no way could I control where I was going. The ocean was my life and I was definitely at the mercy of it. I couldn't move physically or emotionally; I couldn't stretch out and wiggle my toes or drift off into a comfortable sleep. I was totally constricted in every sense.

When the water came up and wet my feet, it relaxed my whole body. I watched the sand crabs running around and digging under the sand. *Can I come, too?*

"Come on, George!" Veronica shouted from farther down the beach. "Let's go!" I hadn't even realized she'd left my side.

It was so hard walking in the sand and water, but it was worth it. I felt free in the breeze as we ventured out farther and farther from the house, from my life. I wasn't feeling pain. The constant piercing pains that hadn't gone away in months were gone. I could see the islands off the shore and the only thing I wanted to do was to rip off my cast and swim to them; maybe not just to the islands, maybe to the end of the world.

I got tired pretty easily and got overheated with the cast. The cool breeze wasn't enough; I had to go deeper in the water. I started to carefully sneak towards the crashing waves.

"George! No, come back," Veronica got frantic when she noticed I was deeper than she was; the ocean is one of her biggest fears.

"I'm fine, you stay there," I said waving her off, staring at my feet disappearing under the water.

"No! Mom said I'm in charge of you and she said to be careful. Does that really seem like you're being careful?" Defiant, she stopped walking.

"I'm not even up to my knees!" I whined; *who would've thought, my little sister giving me orders?*

"Please, I need to stay near you," she pleaded.

"Then you come out here, come on! Sharks can't even get up here, just come on," I waved her over. "It feels so good."

After thinking about it I seemed to have won her over. "You come here first."

I made my way over and we held hands, walking into knee deep water. We walked like that for a couple of minutes; it felt like I was walking on the water. *Could this be my Vienna?*

The next six seconds all seemed to happen at the exact same time.
- One. *Bam*, I felt the shooting pain down my right leg.
- Two. I felt my leg collapsing, just giving up.
- Three. I felt the water splashing up on my face as I fell into the cold Pacific Ocean.
- Four. I heard Veronica scream and felt her arm try to grab me, but miss.
- Five. I took a big gulp of air.
- Six. I took a bigger gulp of water.

I knew I was only in knee-deep water, but it was still shocking. I couldn't get up once I was down there. I was locked in a rigid position underwater and couldn't bend to get up. I wasn't scared while Veronica scrambled to get me out. As the waves went in and out I got plenty of air, I just had to wait for it sometimes.

It wasn't like I was in there for a long time; Veronica helped me up pretty quickly. The reason I wasn't scared, being underwater and not being able to get out, was because I was overcome by sadness.

I was so sad underwater because something as simple as a walk on the beach had turned into another thing that I could not do. When I got up out of the water I was crying, and cried the whole walk back. When I had to tell everyone what happened I just laughed it off like I found it humorous; I didn't.

I felt so pathetic as I limped across the beach and hiked up the stairs to the beach house. I felt embarrassed changing out of my wet clothes and drying my wet hair. I felt sad that my one brief moment of happiness was once again interrupted by pain.

"But I'm not prepared," I argued. "I don't even know what chapter we are on."

"I'm sorry, but the test is today," Mr. Franklin shrugged his shoulders, holding out the test. The shooting pain went down my leg and I bit my lip to hide my agony.

"But I haven't been to the last three classes," I said, getting frustrated.

"I know and we will talk about that list of things for you to do later, but for now you take this test with the rest of the class."

I could tell by his cold stare that he was not budging, so I took the test as politely as I could and waddled to my chair in the corner of the room. I did my half-sit, half-crouch, and wrote my name on the top of the test: *Español 1, Unidad 6.*

What's a "manzana"? I know it's a type of fruit; could it be orange? No that's "naranja;" or is "naranja" the color orange? I knew nothing. *What does all of this mean? If preterite is past tense then what's imperfect? I thought that was past tense, too?*

It was impossible to just show up and be expected to do well on a test when I hadn't even been in class for a week. I was extremely discouraged as I turned in my test – half blank, half scribbles.

My back was killing me and all I wanted to do was to go home. I closed my eyes and tried not to cry. *There is no way I am going to start crying in the middle of class; no way in hell.*

All I could think about was this pain spreading through my lower back as I chewed on my pencil. *How does the first verse of Vienna start?* I had no idea; I couldn't even remember my name the pain was so intense.

"Georgia, are you okay?" Freddy asked me. I opened my eyes to see a couple of people staring and whispering.

"Yeah," I said, trying my best to give a convincing smile. But he was an old friend and teammate, and could tell I wasn't doing well. His comforting hand on my shoulder made me cry even more because these were the first words he had spoken to me in months; the first time he'd even made eye contact with me in months. He'd asked me to the Homecoming dance that year and I declined; there went our friendship.

I didn't know why he decided all of a sudden to comfort me after such a long silence, but that was one of the most interesting parts of this whole thing; realizing which people will step up and who will fall behind. *Who's my real friend?*

I ended up being in so much pain that my friend Evan, who was on the football team and huge, had to carry me down the stairs and to the office where my dad was waiting for me; *talk about being discreet.*

Chapter Eleven

"Have you been wearing it all the time, even to sleep?" Dr. Nine asked me skeptically.

"Yes, I have," I answered.

"She took it off once during a panic attack, but that was it," my dad added.

"You wore it in showers?" he pressed, trying to find the answer to why I was still in pain.

"Yes."

He seemed puzzled and looked down at my file. "Well, the pain shouldn't be bothering you so much."

We waited while he looked everything over and tried to solve this mystery.

"Okay," he started slowly like he wasn't completely sure of what he was going to say. "We are going to stop with the cast." *What!* "We are going to try something else."

"Anything," I said desperately, only to be laughed at by my dad.

"Do you know what a corset is?" he asked, writing on a scrap of paper.

"Like ladies wore in the olden days?" I was confused.

"Yeah, kind of. This one is medical though," he said handing my dad the prescription.

"Why the corset now?" I asked.

"My idea is to still give you the back support, and it should just be like a soft cast to you, but it will only be around your core stomach and back area."

"Are you okay with that?" my dad asked, laughing in the corner.

"More than you will ever know."

My wings had been clipped for too long and now, after months of being stuck on the ground, now I could fly. We shoved the body cast in the trunk of the car (where it stayed for half a year) and when I sat down in the car, *I actually sat down!* For the first time in months I actually sat down, and it felt awesome.

I rolled the window down and my face was actually at a high enough level that I could see out the window. It was like I was seeing the city for the first time. I had been here this whole time, but locked behind walls.

When he brought out the corset I almost laughed, *it's so small!* It was even smaller than I expected and from what I remembered from old movies and such, it would make me look even skinnier.

Okay, when he put it on it didn't make me look any skinnier, but it was a hell of a lot better than the body cast. He put it on tight and I think anyone would have said that it was uncomfortable, but compared to what I was used to, this was fine. *Thank you, Doctor Nine.*

I left there with a new confidence and it followed me all the way home.

"Mom!" I exclaimed as I swung open the front door. She came running in from the kitchen and when she saw me, she stopped.

"What happened?" she asked coming up to me.

"He gave me a corset," I said, pulling up my shirt.

She gave me a hug, my first real hug in weeks and weeks. I had plenty of "hugs" during the body cast, but this hug was different. I could actually feel my mom's tiny body clenched onto mine. I could feel her heart beat and the temperature of her body. There was no longer going to be a wall between other people and me.

When I woke up the next day, all of the excitement was gone. In other words, I was back. So was the pain.

I laid in bed all day feeling sorry for myself. I watched marathons of random shows that I was only half interested in and ate more food than I was actually hungry for. When my mom got home from work she asked me what was up. I wasn't very nice, but instead of walking out of the room offended, my mom kept persisting.

"Why was your day so bad?" she asked.

"Because mom, what would have made it good?" I snapped, "me lying in your bed all day or me sitting up in your bed all day?"

"You don't have to be in bed all day," she said turning down the TV.

"Yes I do, mom," I said giving her a look. "My back was hurting all day!"

"Did you do any art?" she asked calmly.

"No mom, I could barely move."

"I'm gonna take the puppies on a w-a-l-k; wanna come with?" We always had to spell the word out because they learned what "walk" meant.

"Are you kidding me?" I said rudely.

"Come on, don't make me go alone," she pressed. "And besides, it's golden hour."

Those two words made my heart ache; *golden hour.*

"You know there's no golden hour here," I said softly.

"There's always a golden hour," my mom said smiling, "I'll show you where you can see it."

Golden hour is the best time of the day.

We used to live next to Bel-Air, up in the hills that overlook the valley. I grew up in that house, until I was in sixth grade. As a kid, my mom, my sister, and I would always bring our old dog, Cosworth, on walks. We would wait until it got cool outside, but before it got dark, to start our walks.

Since we lived up in the hills, most of the natural scenery was all light brown. The hills by my house weren't grassy, they were mostly dirt. When the sun was just starting to set, it would reflect off the hills and make the whole neighborhood glow under a golden color.

Golden hour was when the mountains that looked ugly during the day could shine, and when dads started to play ball with their sons because they'd just gotten home from work. It was when kids finished their homework and were allowed to play on the jungle gym as a reward, and when a mother could bring her two daughters out on a walk with their dog while dinner was cooking.

Since we'd moved down to the bottom of the hill I hadn't really experienced golden hour in a while, but apparently my mom knew a place. I put on my shoes and hobbled out of the house behind my mom and dogs.

I got out of the gate and I really started to feel my leg and back pain kicking in, but I thought I could push through it. I got half a block and it really started to kill me. By the end of the block I couldn't even cross the street.

"Mom, I have to go back," I said panting.

"Okay, honey."

They walked me back and when I got to the gate they continued their walk. They went to golden hour, I went home.

"Did you see this article?" my grandpa asked, handing me a cutout of a newspaper. "There's a girl playing baseball on a high school team."

"Very cool, grandpa," I said, trying not to look at his forehead. He had been falling a lot late at night and had a couple of nasty cuts on his head.

"You can have this one, I kept it for you," he said smiling.

"Thanks," I put it in my purse.

"How's school going?" he asked, sitting in his armchair. That chair held so many memories.

"Not that well."

"What's the matter? Don't you like it?" He seemed shocked.

"Yeah I do. I just mean that I haven't really been at school a lot."

"I met a man the other day who lives here at the home. He went to Notre Dame High School, the same school you go to. His name's Fred."

"That's cool," I smiled.

"I see you're out of the cast. When am I gonna see you play ball for Notre Dame?"

"I don't know Grandpa, it's not up to me," I was so sick of him asking me that all the time.

"Not up to you? Then who's it up to?"

"I don't know, Grandpa."

"Hang on," he said, getting up and starting to the other room where my grandma was sleeping.

"Wait, let me get your walker." I beat him standing up.

"No," he shooed me to sit back down, but I didn't.

"Grandpa, here," I said dragging it over to him. "You have to use your walker or you're gonna keep hitting your head."

"Ah," he gave me a look, "why would I do that?"

"Why would you do what?"

"Hit my head?" he said, laughing at his own joke. Then he smiled and took the walker from me.

I went and sat in his armchair, the most comfortable chair ever. It was his throne. I heard a noise behind me and turned to see a little hummingbird eating from the feeder on the porch.

I watched the hummingbird and it reminded me of when I'm having a panic attack. Its wings beat as fast as my heart and as blurry as my mind. Hummingbirds were beautiful and delicate, but they were usually alone. I never saw a pack of hummingbirds hanging out together. They were alone like me. Hummingbird wings flapped so fast that it looked like they were flying recklessly at a hundred miles an hour, but in reality they could be going nowhere. It always looked like they worked harder than they had to, which was like me. I felt like everything I had to do, I had to work one hundred times harder than any other kid my age.

My grandpa came back into the room with something in his hand. "Where's your walker?" I asked, clearly frustrated.

"Your grandmother wanted to borrow it," he said smiling.

"Grandma's asleep and can't even get out of bed by herself," I busted him.

"Don't ask me why she wanted it." He handed me the paper in his hand. "Here."

I looked at it and it was a picture of my grandma smiling with a green "Happy New Year" headband on her head; I hadn't seen her smile like that in a while.

"That's New Years," he said smiling and pointing at it. "Look at how beautiful she is."

He was glowing and looked so proud. "Yes Grandpa, she is beautiful."

"Dad, it's getting so much worse," I said one day, limping into his office.

"What is?" he put the TV on mute and looked at me.

"My pain. It's getting hard for me to walk. I am literally walking with a limp, I couldn't even push Grandma's wheelchair to take her on a walk."

"Well, what can we do?" he asked helplessly.

"I don't know, dad. I don't know."

"Do you think the corset is working?"

"No, I don't."

"Well, you have an appointment with an important doctor at a big children's hospital next week, and we are on the waiting list for the UCLA Pediatric Pain Management Clinic. What else do you think we can do?"

"I don't know, dad."

"Do you want to call Dr. Nine?"

"No, he doesn't help. This corset doesn't help and neither did the cast." I started to take it off.

"Now we don't know that," he said, putting his hand up to stop me.

"Yes we do!" I snapped, clearly irritated. "These casts have done nothing but embarrass me and make my life a living hell!"

He thought for a moment and then shrugged, "Okay, if you don't think it helps, then take it off."

The next doctor's office was on the top floor of an extremely tall building. I remember whenever someone would take the elevator all the way up, the whole building would shake and scare the hell out of me.

Doctor Eleven was a pediatric neurosurgeon so the waiting room was full of kids with disabilities. It was heartbreaking and a little uncomfortable when I seemed to be the only person who wasn't in a wheelchair staring into space, or didn't have a helmet on. After a while these beautiful little kids would come up to me and my dad and just look at us. It made me realize that what I had might not be so bad after all; plenty of people have it a lot worse.

Since the waiting room was so full there were literally no empty chairs; my dad and I had to stand. Whenever I stood for too long I would get dizzy and my pains would get worse, but that's what we had to do. They will be with us as soon as possible.

You've got your passion, you've got your pride
but don't you know that only fools are satisfied?
Dream on, but don't imagine they'll all come true
When will you realize, Vienna waits for you?

No Billy, I <u>had</u> my passion and I <u>had</u> my pride; I don't have it anymore. Fools are satisfied but fools can also be unsatisfied, too, since I am a fool. I am a fool for having to ask other people what's wrong with me rather than knowing on my own. "Dream on;" dream on to what Billy? I have been dreaming constantly and about the smallest things. I have been dreaming about being able to run a lap around the track at my school and I have been dreaming to go see a movie with my friends; I'm not asking for much. Oh I wouldn't dare "imagine they'll all come true," wouldn't ever expect that much out of my sucky life. Vienna doesn't exist, at least not for me anyway.

"I just don't see anything wrong in any of these," Dr. Eleven said looking through my manila envelopes. *Come on, Dr. Eleven. Be my hero.*

"Do you see the pars defect that Dr. Nine saw?" my dad asked.

"Yes," he nodded still looking down, "I see that, but it shouldn't be causing her this much pain."

"Then what is?" my dad was clearly frustrated.

"I'm just not sure, Mr. Huston, I'm sorry."

I left there as deflated as could be; going down that long elevator was ironic because that's how far down my heart was falling as well.

When we got to the parking lot I started sobbing. I couldn't hold it in anymore.

"What's going on?" I whined to my dad as we got in the car. I was in my school uniform but I was not going to school that day.

"I don't know, Georgia," my dad said, pausing to think before he started the car.

"I'm in so much pain right now," I said throwing my head back.

"Why didn't you tell the doctor that? We were just in with a doctor." He was clearly irritated pulling out of the parking lot into downtown L.A. traffic.

"It wouldn't have made a difference. He didn't know, just like everyone else."

"You can't wait until we are in the car to start talking about how much pain you're in."

"Okay, dad."

"Are you going to school today?"

"No dad, I can't. I can barely walk," I was getting really mad.

"Okay, that's fine but you've got to start telling the doctors how much pain you're in."

"I will, dad," I snapped.

"When have I heard that before?" he muttered under his breath.

Chapter Twelve

After a couple of minutes of silence I just had to ask.

"Dad," I took a deep breath. "Am I crazy?"

Immediately his mood shifted and he gave me the most sincere look. "No, you're not."

"Yes I am, dad. Why are you still pretending?"

"I'm not pretending. Why would I pretend about that? Why would I lie to you about that?"

"I don't know, but you are. I know what the doctors all ask you when they have me leave the room. They ask if I'm making it up to get attention, I know they are," I said, getting worked up in my emotions.

"Sometimes they do, yeah," he said lightly, looking at the road, "but do you know what I say every time?"

"I'm not in the room," I said bluntly.

"Well," he started, "I look them in the eye and I ask them why they think you would make this up. I ask them if anyone they know would rather be sitting in doctors' waiting rooms than out with friends. I ask them what kid would stop playing sports and trade cleats for a body cast. And then I stop asking and I tell them that if they really knew you, they wouldn't need to ask. They would already know that there is no way anyone, especially not you, would make all of this up to get attention."

I started crying harder, "But what if I am making this up?"

"You're not."

"How would *you* know?"

"Because I know you."

"But the fact that I'm not making this up just proves that I *am* crazy; that something *is* wrong with me."

"No it doesn't," he said as calmly and matter-of-factly as could be. "Why does it have to mean that?"

"Because no doctor can find it, so it's all my head."

"Just because no doctor has found it yet doesn't mean it's not there."

"How are you so sure? If I say that I'm crazy then I am, because I know myself better than anyone."

"Then you must not know yourself that well."

My dad had an old friend who was a neurologist, so we thought we'd give him a try. I didn't exactly know what a neurologist was, but I thought that maybe since he knew my dad, he would give us a little more attention and a little better advice.

His office was about an hour and a half away, but with traffic it took almost two. When I was led into my exam room I noticed a lot of outlines of people on the walls, but instead of bones there were lines going everywhere; nerves. I was used to seeing bones on the chart figures since all the doctors that I'd seen were bone guys. *Maybe that's a good sign, maybe we need a new point of view. Oh this guy is going to be it.... Dr. Twelve, be my hero.*

"Jimmy!" In came Dr. Twelve with a glowing smile and they immediately shook hands. "Good to see you!"

"You too," my dad greeted him. "This is my daughter, Georgia."

"Well, hey there," he said shaking my hand, still smiling.

"Hi," I responded.

He looked at my dad and then down at my chart. "Now I know we spoke a bit on the phone, but can you just give me a little background to remind me?"

"Oh yeah, sure…" And there he went, like he had rehearsed it over and over again. He knew his script flawlessly because he *had* been rehearsing it over and over again. Every time we saw a new doctor he would have to repeat the same exact story but, every time we saw a new doctor that meant that a past doctor had failed, so he would have to add something about them, too. The story kept growing and getting longer to the point where I would just tune it out.

Dr. Twelve was the first of all the doctors who seemed to be genuinely hanging onto every word. He was different, *I can feel it.*

"So you're hoping that – well, not hoping – but the reason you came to me is that you think it might not have to do with her skeleton, but with her nervous system?" Dr. Twelve asked thoughtfully.

"Yes, because no one else can find it," my dad always got really passionate when trying to explain what we were going through with someone new. "We are going to the best doctors in the state, and they can't find it!"

"I understand," Dr. Twelve said sympathetically. "Let's see if we can."

He took out of his pocket a small red object. It looked like a game piece from the board game "Sorry." *How ironic, that's what all the doctors end up telling me.* This was slightly different from one of the game pieces though, in that at the bottom, it had a tiny needle-like thing coming out of it. *Needle?!*

"What is that?" I asked, putting my hand in between me and the needle.

"This?" he grinned, holding it up, "this is just a tool I use to see where your most sensitive areas are."

"But I *know* where my most sensitive areas are. I can just tell you."

"Sometimes when I press on the nerves with this, we find new information."

"Like what?" I asked bluntly, "do you think my foot hurts and I just don't know it, but this red thing is going to show you that it does?"

"No, I just want to see for myself where you're hurting." He took my hand, "And feel, this doesn't even hurt, it's not that sharp."

I pulled my hand away, "I don't like needles."

"Look," he laughed and started poking himself in the hand with it. I looked at his face to see if there was any pain, but I couldn't see any. I took it from him and felt the tip with my finger; *it's really not that sharp.*

When I gave him the "all clear" he proceeded. He took the red poker and started at my right hand, working his way up my arm. The poking gave me a little discomfort, but nothing worth mentioning. He poked around my neck, which tickled a little bit; it was hard not to cringe. He crossed over and went down my left arm to my hand; still nothing unusual. He went down the side of my left ribs, down the outside of my leg and to my foot. He prodded the bottom of my foot which didn't tickle or hurt, it just didn't feel good. He nudged it up the inside of my left leg and then crossed over to the inside of my right leg. When he got to the outside of my right leg, it started getting extremely sensitive.

"There," I said with my eyes closed as he got to the middle of the outside of my right thigh. He kept going up my leg and up my right ribs without saying a word.

"Can you turn around?" he asked when he got to my armpit area. *Uh oh, time for the back.* I was dreading that.

He lightly stabbed all over my back, literally *all over.* I told him where it hurt and where it didn't hurt and when he put that little red game piece in his coat pocket I was so relieved.

"Did she pass?" my dad joked.

For the first time since I'd met him, Dr. Twelve looked serious. "The only advice that I can give you is to take a nerve test that I can order for you."

"Okay, then we'll do that," my dad said.

"Well, it's all about needles," he said looking at me.

"No," I shook my head.

"What's the test?" My dad put his hand up to tell me to stop.

"They would put needles all over your body and try to stimulate your nerves. It's not fun."

"Is there any other kind of test?" I begged.

Another doctor who threw up his hands. *Will this ever end?*

We were desperate, so I had to suck it up and take the stupid test.

I can remember that office and those people more clearly than anything else in that time period. I remember the dimly lit hallway of the big office building and walking into the waiting room, which was so big but so empty. I remember the big plants in all the corners of the room and I could tell by the light coming in through the blinds that it was golden hour.

A lady who looked like my eighth grade social studies teacher came out and introduced herself. I was so nervous I don't even remember any of the conversation. She brought me into the back and took me into the first room on the right. I sat down and there was a huge computer screen across from me.

She left for a moment and when she came back there was another lady with her, a pre-med student who was going to be observing today's "procedure." *Awesome.*

They asked me questions about *everything*. They asked if I was unhappy; I said "yes." They asked if I was depressed; I said, "I think so." They asked if I was suicidal; I said "no." It went on like that for a while.

There were personal questions, too, that required a lot of detail. But, I obeyed; *who knows, this might work. Come on ladies, be my heros.*

After what seemed like forever they brought me into another room that looked a lot more intimidating than the first. It was very bright, which made me uncomfortable; I am very sensitive to light.

There were a number of monitors, all facing a desk and chair. There was a bed-like thing that they told me to lie on; *Umm, no thanks.* I was so scared I didn't even know what was going on. I was in a gown and before I knew it, I was having needles stuck into my body.

The needles were all attached to long wires that went to the monitors. I heard a lot of noises; clicking, tapping, and buzzing. I felt pulling, sticking, and pinching. I tried to take myself somewhere else, anywhere but there.

It was no surprise when the test didn't find anything. I was getting pretty disenchanted with doctors at this point.

I'm somewhere on a tropical beach, these aren't needles – it's the breeze that I feel on my skin. That's not clicking, those are the waves. I'm not sweating because I'm scared; it's because of the warm sun on my back.

I knew not all doctors were bad, that was just an unfortunate recurring theme for me. We also had some extraordinary doctors help us, even though we never met them.

Jenny's mom, Pam, had a friend who became Dr. Thirteen and generously consulted with my dad over the phone. He was a big help because he was impartial and knew a lot about pain, guiding us away from places that would only be giving me more drugs. He went out of his way to help us even though he didn't even know me.

My dad found Dr. Fourteen, an orthopedic surgeon, through his racing friends. We didn't know him personally but my dad spent hours on the phone telling him my story. He didn't know us at all, but he listened and gave advice. My dad would ask what we were doing wrong or if there was anything more we could do; he was even willing to take me up to San Francisco to see Dr. Fourteen. He said, "No, you're going to the best minds in California, You're doing all the right things, you've just got to keep going." Even though he told my dad we were doing everything right, it was hard for us to see it that way at the time.

Russ had surgery for a herniated disc during all my problems. His surgery went well and when he went back to his orthopedic surgeon, he brought my MRIs and X-rays with him to show Dr. Sixteen. Though he couldn't figure out what was wrong, he did help us eliminate an alarming diagnosis that had been suggested.

All of these doctors gave us guidance without meeting or talking to me and we were extremely grateful for their generosity and counsel.

Slow down, you crazy child
you're so ambitious for a juvenile

*But then if you're so smart, tell me
Why are you still so afraid?*

Slow down; slow – sluggish, inactive, lazy; down – depressed, miserable, dejected. Crazy child; crazy means foolish, unwise, and senseless. Child means immature. How can I be ambitious? I have nothing to work towards. I'm not smart, just look at my grades; I'm pretty sure I am failing out of school. Why am I still so afraid; afraid means anxious, terrified, and petrified. What's not to be anxious of? Terrified of? Petrified of?

"Let's play a board game," Jenny suggested, walking to my closet.

"Okay." I really didn't care what we did; I was so tired.

"Hmm," she said looking in my closet at the board games I had. I hadn't played a board game in forever; I didn't even know which ones I had. "Trouble?"

"No, people always get into fights over that game."

"Life?"

"Too easy."

"Monopoly?"

I shrugged, "Okay."

She was the thimble, I was the shoe, and the board was our world. We played that game for hours and that started my Monopoly obsession. I became a master at Monopoly and would want to play it twenty-four/seven. I didn't care who it was or what mood they were in, if someone came into the house, I would ask them to play Monopoly with me.

Something between the game and me just clicked. It was like my alter ego where I could do whatever I wanted. I could go out and buy as many properties as I wanted. I could make deals with my properties to get more properties. I could double the rent or put as many houses on it as I wanted. I could knock people out of the game just by their landing on my nasty properties once. Monopoly was mine; all mine.

My dad opened the door, "Okay, Jenny, your mom just called; she wants you home."

"Did she say why she wanted me home so early?" Jenny asked.

"Yeah, your grandparents are coming over for dinner."

"I thought they were coming tomorrow night."

"I'm just telling you what she told me."

"Okay, I'll be right out."

Jenny got all her things together while I cleaned up the Monopoly board game. As I picked my hotels and her houses off the board I felt sad, like I was taking away the life that I wanted. It's not that I wanted to be successful in real estate when I was older; I just wanted to be successful. I wanted to have the power to do whatever I wanted; *who wouldn't?*

With every game piece I took off the board, I was brought back to the reality that I couldn't do whatever I wanted; I couldn't really do anything I wanted. As I stacked the money back into the box I felt my pain starting to come back. It became clear to me at that moment that Monopoly was my escape from pain – and from the pain of being me.

Chapter Thirteen

Jenny lived in Woodland Hills, so the car ride from my house was about twenty minutes on a good day. My dad was driving, I was sitting in the front seat, and Jenny was in the back.

A couple of minutes went by in silence. I was looking out the window, spacing, and thinking about my life. *What was going to happen to my grades? Would I have to repeat my ninth grade year or just second semester?*

I thought about my friends and how soccer season was over, but I hadn't even played in one game. I thought about the fact that I barely knew any Spanish or how to write a thesis statement. I didn't know any of the foundations for the subjects that I would have to study for the rest of my high school career. I was in way over my head and I knew it. I thought about what everyone at school would say about me; *where do they think I am?*

How did we get here? It seemed that in the blink of an eye we had traveled two freeway exits. *How is that possible? Did I fall asleep? No, I couldn't have – I'm not tired.*

I looked over at my dad, who was giving me a weird look. "Did you fall asleep?" my dad asked.

"I guess."

I really had no idea, but that had to be the only explanation. I continued looking out the window and thinking.

We passed the Balboa exit. If we were to exit, there would be a fork in the road. If you turn left, you get to my doctor's office; if you turn right you go to the park where I played soccer for years. I used to be at a fork in my life and I turned right. I turned in the direction of my bright future and what made me happy, but somehow I'd accidently made a U-turn and ended up at the doctor's office. No more U-turns anymore. I've found my destination, *this is my life.*

How are we already exiting at Winnetka? We were just at Balboa! What's going on?

"Georgia, what happened?" my dad asked, alarmed. Both he and Jenny were eyeing me intently.

"I don't know," I said concentrating, trying to figure out anything that could remind me of what had happened. *Where did I go?*

"Did you pass out?" he asked.

"I don't know, dad!" I was getting really frustrated.

"I just want to know what happened."

"So do I!" I snapped.

The only time I had ever passed out was at my thirteenth birthday party. It was an ice skating party and while we were setting up I passed out cold on the floor for a couple of seconds. When I woke up I had no idea what had happened, and we never really figured out what happened or why. Coincidentally, Jenny was the only other person in the room when I passed out then, too. *"Too?" So did I pass out?*

"When's my appointment at the UCLA pain thing?"

"It's in a while, Georgia," my dad answered somberly.

"How long?" I pressed.

"We don't know the exact date," he kept avoiding it.

"What did they say?"

"Six months," he said looking away from me. *Six months!*

"What am I going to do for another six months," I moaned. "Dad, I can't do this for another six months. I really can't."

"I know Georgia, I can't either. But I don't know if it will even be that helpful."

"What do you mean?" This was the first time I'd heard this.

"It's the UCLA Pediatric Pain Management Clinic. That name means it's a last resort, when you don't have any more options. It's for learning how to live with the pain, to *manage* it."

"So then why are we waiting for it? Have you given up?"

"No, Georgia. I haven't given up and neither have you."

As I was watching TV one day I got a text from an old friend I hadn't talked to in almost a year. Ella was my close friend from middle school, but after we'd graduated we hadn't been in touch.

Ella: Georgia!! Whatsup! I miss uuuu
Me: Hey! Nothing really just watching tv

Ella: What have u been up 2
Me: Just hanging out hbu
Ella: Ya same same. Just enjoying high school

We texted for a while before I decided to tell her the truth. I thought about having her keep thinking that I was cool and having fun like she was, but then I decided *what do I have to lose? I never see her anyway.*

It was hard to tell her everything at first. It was the first time that I was telling the story rather than my dad. It was weird hearing it from my point of view, with my thoughts and feelings, but after a while it became surprisingly easy and I just poured everything out to her. Mind you it was just over text, but it was extremely relieving.

While I wrote, she read. She asked questions, she sympathized; she cared. By the end of the night she asked if she could come over to see me. I didn't want her to; I didn't want anyone to see me. My embarrassment at my situation ate away at me as much as the pain did. *Would she even recognize me if she came over? Would she even like me anymore?*

My mom was lying in bed next to me, so I told her that Ella wanted to visit. I couldn't see her face in the darkness, but I could feel her mood change.

"Yes! When does she want to come?" she asked, clearly excited.

"I don't know yet. She just asked if she could."

"Well, tell her 'yes.'"

"But I don't know if I want her to or not," I whined.

"Why not, Peaches? She wants to see you."

"No, she doesn't. She wants to see who I used to be – who she remembers me as."

"George, that's still you. You are the same person," she said, turning the TV off to get my attention.

"No, it's not."

"Invite her over, honey. What do you have to lose?"

"She won't like me anymore."

"You don't know that. Invite her over."

"But mom, I can't do anything. What are we gonna do, just lie in bed and watch a movie? That won't be fun for her, I promise you."

"Ask her. Let her make the decision."

Ella wanted to come. She said she didn't care what we did; she just wanted to see me.

She was coming over in two days.

"Are you going to school today?" my dad asked, turning on the light to wake me up.

The light burned through my eyes. "No, I can't today, dad." Not only was I in pain and got little sleep, I was afraid of school. School had become my enemy that haunted almost all of my thoughts. It depressed me and gave me major anxiety.

It was 11:17 when I woke up in my parents' room; what seemed like my new room. I turned on the TV and put on a TLC show, "Say Yes to the Dress." It's about future brides shopping for lavish wedding dresses and having fun with their friends, all looking forward to the big day. *I'm never going to have a day like that, am I?*

Who's this bride; where'd the blonde one go? I re-wound the show back a couple of minutes until I found the blonde bride that I'd remembered. *How did it get to this new bride so fast?* Then my heart sank as I started to realize the possibilities. *Could I have passed out again?*

No, I couldn't have. I don't do that. How could I pass out and not know it?

I began to cry lightly to myself; *what's going on?*

My heart started to race while I reflected back on the past couple of weeks. *Could I have been passing out this whole time and just not noticed? What have I missed?*

I felt light-headed and I saw spots. I cried out and grabbed my back as the pain stabbed my spine. *Why is this happening to me?*

I can't breathe, I can't breathe. My eyes got wide and I lost my train of thought. The room got really dark for two seconds, and then went back to its normal lighting. I was sweating but couldn't stand up to turn on the fan. The TV volume got really loud all of a sudden and stayed loud. *The remote's all the way over there, how does it keep getting louder?*

I'm crazy, none of this is really happening – you're crazy, Georgia. They are going to lock you up and visit you every other Thursday for the rest of your life. You won't have to worry about outfits anymore, you'll be in a strait jacket.

This can't be me, I can't be crazy.

But I am.

But I don't hear phantom voices, I don't see hallucinations. Crazy people see and hear things.

That's not the only way to be crazy.

Every thought that went through my head was immediately contradicted.

My family would visit me more than every other Thursday, they love me.

How would I even know if they visited me or not? I probably won't recognize them anymore.

"I can't, I can't!" I shouted at my dad. *When did he get in here?*

"But you have to, honey. Please," he pleaded with me. I had never heard his voice like that. *I have to what? What was he asking me to do?*

Am I dying?

I can't feel my body, am I watching this happen from somewhere else?

"No, b-but Dad-d I d-don't want that," I cried out. *What was I saying?*

My mind was in a different place but I had no idea where. I was answering questions and having a full conversation with my dad that I had no recollection of. I was like a robot just spitting out answers, but there was nothing behind them. *What is going on?*

Where am I? Am I on a cloud?

I'm drowning.

"Should I?" My dad's voice echoed in my ear.

How am I under water? Where'd the cloud go?!

"Georgia, I need to know. Should I or not?"

This is like a dream I had once. I was on a sinking ship, but the only one on it. I could feel the boat sinking deeper and deeper into the ocean. I was inside the boat, trapped by a window. I could see the water rising and sky disappearing. The air was getting thicker and I knew I was going to die. I was going to die alone – will anyone know how I died?

"Yes, I need an ambulance for my daughter, please."

Did I tell anyone I was going on this ship? Will they find me at the bottom of the ocean or will I stay down there forever? I felt the cold water trickling down the walls and falling to my feet.

"She's fourteen. Please...."

I looked up as I felt the water rising to my knees. I looked up and I saw my dad looking down at me. He was looking down through the window, *what was he doing out there?* The water was at my waist and I started to get tired. I stared into my dad's eyes and wanted to ask him why he wasn't opening the window, why he wasn't letting me out.

I could see my big red puffy eyes in the reflection of the window. I could see my tears falling down my cheeks and my lip start to quiver. I could see me take off my glasses and rub my swollen eyes.

"Let me out dad, the water's cold," I cried out to him.

He just looked at me, was this still my dream or was this really happening? My heart stopped, *I don't have glasses.*

Wake up Georgia, wake up. I scratched at my arms, *wake up.* My dad reached through the window and pulled my arms away. *Why didn't any water get through when he did that?*

The water was so cold and almost to my shoulders, my chattering teeth and shivering body were all going at the same fast pace. *That wasn't my reflection.*

"I have to go open the gate for the paramedics – don't move," my dad said holding my shoulders. "Promise me Georgia, you won't move." I had never heard pleading that desperate in my life.

"Dad!" I shouted with my mouth to the window. *Where's he going? Is he leaving me here to drown?*

If that wasn't my reflection crying, then who was it?

"Georgia, keep talking to me, honey." *Where is that voice coming from?*

"Georgia." *How does he know my name?*

"They're almost there, Georgia. Calm down. You have to calm down." *But I don't know you, how'd you get in my house?*

Who was crying behind me when I thought it was my reflection? Who else was on the boat with me?

The man talking to me was coming through the telephone next to my ear. *I'm gonna lose him once I go under the water.*

I can't breathe –

"I can't breathe!"

Somebody help me.

"Somebody help me!"

"We're going to help you, Georgia. I am your 911 operator, remember? I am here to help you."

The water is up to my neck, I have to stand on my toes to breathe.

My dad's face came back into the window, I can see him. I can see him, and now the reflections of my puffy eyes are back.

I'm under water.

I never got to take my last gulp of air, I wasn't ready.

Open the window, dad.

Open it.

Just as my eyes were closing, closing for good, the window opened and tons of hands came in. They all went straight for me and grabbed me all over my body. I still couldn't breathe but they pulled me out anyway. They swam with me up to where the sky meets the sea and threw me out. I couldn't move any part of my body, everything was cramped.

They pulled me up and strapped me onto their raft. *I still don't feel safe. Get me out of here.* One man pushed the raft from behind and the other pulled it. The ocean was really rocky and my body was flopping around. *Please don't let me fall back in, I can't swim right now. Please, please don't let me fall.*

Is one of the men on the boat singing? Why are they making a joke out of this? They are making siren noises, stop playing around!

Wait! Turn around; there was someone else on the boat with me. I saw them when I was looking through the window. It couldn't have been my reflection, I know that now. Someone's still there! Someone was on the sinking boat with me! Someone needs help!

When they got me to the shore I could feel them pull my raft up onto the sand. I felt the strong arms carefully pick me up and put me gently down back on the cloud. They wished me luck and the voices were gone. *Am I in heaven?*

The last place I would ever go is heaven. Have I not seen all the torture I have been inflicting on my loved ones for months? I don't deserve to be saved, I don't deserve to go to heaven.

I don't even know what heaven is. Heaven is supposed to be a happy place where everyone feels wonderful. I don't even know how to feel that way, all I know is suffering – all I know is pain.

Who did I leave on the boat? Who is still there sinking?

Another reason why I don't deserve to go to heaven, I don't deserve this cloud.

Who was the person crying with the glasses? I only saw them when I could see my dad through the window.

Where am I now?

Am I in a coma?

My dad has glasses.

What is that noise?

But dad never cries; I have literally never seen him cry. He doesn't cry.

Who's drowning on the boat while I am up on the cloud?

Who am I letting drown?

My dad has glasses.

I was surprised when Dr. Nine agreed to let me stop wearing the corset. He seemed to understand the stress it caused and he believed that I had real pain.

But then he said, "I would like Georgia to get an epidural today. They do them at the Tarzana hospital."

"Isn't that what pregnant people get?" I asked, hoping I didn't sound too stupid.

"Yes," Dr. Nine nodded, "that is one of the uses, but there are many more. Another use is to relieve back pain."

My dad looked distressed, "I don't want her to get an epidural."

"It will stop her pain," Dr. Nine insisted.

"Until it wears off. What then?"

Dr. Nine got mad at my dad. "Do you want her to keep suffering?"

"No, that's the last thing we want. I just don't feel comfortable having my fourteen-year-old daughter get an epidural."

"Then I don't know what to tell you," Dr. Nine answered.

But he gave us another prescription for pills – stronger pills that I didn't want.

"Can I draw you?" I asked my sister.

"Fine," she said sitting down on the bed, "but, I get to pick what channel we watch."

"Deal."

She doesn't look like a little kid anymore. She's so beautiful, how did she get this beautiful?

I took a dark pencil and I drew her big green eyes, opened as wide as they could be since she was watching TV. I drew her light blonde eyebrows that angularly shaped her facial expressions. I drew her big, kissy lips slightly opened like she was shocked. Her hair was swept away from her face and I shaded all the dark spots with my finger. I darkened around the outside of her head to give it some depth and I was done. *She looks so much older. She looks so beautiful.*

"Thanks." I put my sketchbook down.

"You're welcome," her eyes were glued to the TV.

"Veronica, can I ask you for a favor?"

"Depends on what it is."

"Can you give me a massage?"

"Where?" still looking at the TV.

"My back. Please, Nakks."

"Fine."

I started texting my friends more since I was in a happier mood lately. Raquel and Solene kept asking if they could come over and see me, but I kept making up excuses. I wasn't ready for my school friends to see what I was really going through. I wanted them to remember me as I used to be; when I was fun.

"I'll buy it." I was determined to buy every property I could land on.
"Come on, let me get the greens. You have the two blues," Jenny begged.
I laughed, "Sorry."
"I'm thirsty, I'll be right back."
"Get me something, too," I begged as she walked out of her room.
I looked down and smiled at my stack of money. *How much do I have? One hundred, one hundred and twenty...*

I opened my eyes and for some reason my head was on the carpet. I sat up and saw Jenny sitting on her bed looking at me. She looked absolutely horrified and that's when I knew that I had just passed out.
The last thing I ever wanted was for my friends to see me passed out; *how embarrassing.*
"Come on, it's your turn." I tried to play it off like nothing had happened, but she still had the shocked expression on her face. *How long was I out? How long was she there?*

One more week, one more week until UCLA. One more week of pain.
I dreamed about what my life would be like without pain; *it's going to be amazing.*

"Hey Sare Sare," I smiled and gave her a huge hug.
"Thank you so much for doing this," Dawn said, handing Sarah's sleepover bag to my mom.
"Not a problem at all," my mom said.
"I put her car seat on the porch and I should be back sometime tomorrow. I'm sorry I can't stay. I'm late." She hugged us all goodbye and she was gone.
"Can we play in your room?" Sarah asked looking up at me.
I smiled, "Yes." I got up and started out of the room.
She ran after me, "What happened to your leg?"
"It's just been hurting lately, but I'm okay."
"Cause of your back? Like Talia?"

"Yeah, because of my back." I sat down on my bed. "Can you close the door, please? Thanks, baby."

"Can I play with your bear?" she asked holding up one of my stuffed animals.

"Yes, you may."

"I be the bear, you be the dog," she said handing me a small dog.

"Okay Sarah."

"Bear's name is Andre, what's yours?"

I smiled. Andre was her little boyfriend at the time. "My dog's name is Sarah."

"No," she laughed, "I'm Sarah."

"No, your name is Andre."

"For real I'm Sarah," she argued.

"Nope, you're Andre."

Owe.

"Auntie Nin!"

I opened my eyes and I was lying on the floor of my room. *Did I fall off my bed?*

"Auntie Nin!"

I sat up and I saw Sarah's wide eyes looking at me. She looked so scared and confused; *what does she think happened?*

"Sorry Sarah," I said ashamed.

"Did you go night night?" she asked curiously.

"Yes, Sarah. I went night night."

"Mommy said you sometimes go night night when it's day."

"Unfortunately your Mommy's right."

> *Raquel: Hey! Whatsup*
> *Me: Nothing just watching TV*
> *Raquel: When can Solene and I come over?*
> *Me: Idk I have to ask my parents.*
> *Raquel: How bout on Wednesday?*
> *Me: I'll let you know*

I didn't have to ask my parents. I knew that they would be for it. I was so conflicted because on one hand it could be like when Ella came over, on the other it could backfire and be awful for them. *I'm doing them a favor by not letting them come over. It would be a waste of their time. I'm saying 'no' for their sakes.*

Chapter Fifteen

What am I going to do about school? I'm failing my freshman year. Am I ever going to graduate? All my friends will be going off to college while I just stay here and rot.

Oh no. I felt the rush of blood shoot into my brain. I felt my heartbeat increasing. I saw the spots and I felt the pain in my leg.

"Dad!" I shouted, "Dad!"

I heard him get out of his chair and run down the hallway. "What is it?" he yelled.

"I'm having another panic attack," I mumbled through a clenched jaw, my eyes shut tight.

"Oh God," he said sitting down on the bed next to me. "What can I do?"

"I don't know, dad."

"What do you need? I'll get you anything." I could hear how desperately he was asking, but I didn't have an answer for him.

"Washcloth," I said, partly so he could feel like he was helping. *I don't want to go through this again.*

I put the washcloth over my face and tried to take deep breaths; *why is this happening to me?*

"Here's some medicine that Dr. Nine said to take during your panic attacks. It's going to relax you." I took it.

He sat there with me, helplessly watching. *I'm a good girl; I don't drink, I don't do drugs, I don't even lie! So why me?*

"Georgia, Veronica gets out of school in half an hour," he said softly, his eyes anxiously flickering back and forth between the clock on the wall and me.

"T-that's fine, this-s is-isn't ev-ven a b-bad one."

"I can't leave you like this."

"Y-yes you c-can. G-get Ver-r-ronica."

"I'm going to call Jaron and see if he can get her."

Jaron was my dad's close friend and old writing buddy. He was an interesting man with a quirky sense of humor, but he was a good guy and I used to go to lunch with him all the time. He had been in my life for as long as I could remember.

He said he could pick up Veronica so my dad could stay with me. I was going crazy and my dad didn't know what to do. He looked so confused and lost, he was breaking down.

He was acting differently this time, he seemed so overwhelmed. It wasn't that bad an attack, I think it was just the straw that broke the camel's back and he needed help.

"I need to make a call," and he left the room.

What am I doing to my poor dad?

He came back in. "Christiana and Azmi are coming over."

Christiana and Azmi's family had been our friends since Veronica and their oldest son were in pre-school together. I often babysat for them before all this happened, and they only lived a few blocks away. Azmi was a heart surgeon, so I think my dad called him for that reason; because he was a doctor and my dad didn't know what to do. We needed a doctor we could trust.

"Hey, Georgia." I heard Azmi's voice so I opened my eyes.

I smiled, "H-hi."

Christiana sat down on the bed right next to my shaking body and whipped my wet hair out of my eyes. Everything on my face was wet from my tears and sweat. "Calm down, Georgia."

"I c-c-can't," I shook my head.

"Take deep breaths, you can do it," Azmi said.

My dad popped his head in. "Where did the dogs go?"

"I haven't seen them," Azmi said, looking around.

My dad left for a moment and came back. "Did you guys close the gate?"

"Oh no, I don't think so," Christiana said sitting up.

Azmi and my dad chased my dogs down the street while Christiana comforted me. It was pretty chaotic.

That support from other people meant the world to me and together we got through it. It was such a humbling experience to feel so cared for by people, besides my family, who went out of their way to help me.

Poor Veronica, waiting there late after school, wondering where Dad was. She was probably the last one sitting on the school lawn. *I feel awful.*

Who am I to get all of the attention? What about Veronica?

She is so nice to me; she has really stepped up. She makes me food when I'm hungry, she rubs my back when it hurts; she even does my chores for me.

She misses homework assignments because I ask her to lie with me for another ten minutes over and over. I love her company, but I'm just being selfish. She has her own life, her own problems to worry about.

How does she feel about all this?

"But I don't think I can walk on my leg today."

"You have to, Georgia," my mom replied.

"Can we use grandma's wheelchair?" I asked with big, puppy dog eyes. I really could not imagine walking on my leg, it hurt so badly.

"No honey, we can't." She gently put my hair behind my ear. "What about your crutches?"

I was not excited to see those things come out of my closet again. I never wanted to have to use crutches again, but I'd been doing a lot of things I didn't want to do lately.

It took us a lot longer for me to get everywhere when I was using crutches, but every time I attempted to put weight on my right leg it throbbed even more.

"Are you sure you can walk back? I can go get the car and pick you up," Jojo offered.

"No, I'm fine. Really." I was already mortified after passing out at the table. My dad and I had gone out to lunch with Jojo and Sean at a really nice restaurant, but I passed out and my dad caught my face just before it went into my plate.

It was a beautiful day outside as the four of us made our way down the block. I saw a hummingbird flying around a bird feeder at a nearby house and thought of my grandparents.

I was going as fast as I could on the crutches, trying to keep up with a hyper four-year-old boy. My eyes were glued to the concrete sidewalk as I concentrated on every hop so that I wouldn't fall. I was humming "Vienna" to myself and smelling the beautiful gardens as we passed.

I felt Jojo's delicate hand rubbing on my back and hot concrete on my face; *not again.*

"Are you okay?" my dad asked.

No! "Yeah, I'm fine."

I sat up and pretended like nothing happened again, but I was in a lot of pain. I'd scratched up my elbows and knees; I also hit my head when I fell.

I actually passed out while I was walking on my crutches, which scared the hell out of me. That meant that I wasn't always going to pass out in the comfort of my parents' bed or where my dad could catch me. I felt like I was in danger; *should I even be allowed out of the house?*

"Mom!"

I heard running from across the house, "I'm coming! I'm coming!"

When she swung the door open she looked very nervous.

"What is it?"

"It hurts to move," I said crying lightly.

"Jimmy!" she called.

"What is it?" My dad came in.

"She says it hurts to move," mom explained worriedly.

"Do you want some medicine?"

"No," the thought of that made me cry even more. "No more medicine," I pleaded.

"Okay, okay, it's just an option," he said defensively.

"No medicine today, promise me that."

"If you need it...."

"Promise me? Please?"

"Okay, no medicine," and he left.

"Mommy," I pleaded, "can you stay with me, please?"

"Yes, honey."

We had a number of different movies on the TV during that day, but didn't watch any of them. That Sunday was horrible and all I was thinking about all day was that my UCLA appointment was the next day.

I barely moved that day and I didn't eat either. There is nothing that I wanted more than pain relief, *but don't worry, it's coming tomorrow.* My mom didn't move from my side that day.

She held me and wiped my tears like she had done my whole life. She had always been there for me in a way that no one else was. She was supportive in a way that no one else was. She had a way of just being there and not needing to do anything. Her presence made all the difference when I was in pain.

I loved the way when she would hug me, her huge hair would suffocate me. I loved the way whenever I would stand up she would tell me how she thought I'd grown. I loved how every day she would call me a new nickname and that she was always there for me to draw, beat at Monopoly, or just hold. Whatever I needed, she was there and always will be.

"I can't do this, Mommy." I buried my face in her chest.

"Yes you can, honey. Everything's going to be okay." She kissed my hair.

"No, it's not Mommy, it hurts."

"I know, baby. But tomorrow is your appointment and everything is going to be okay. Just hang on until tomorrow."

Tomorrow.

> *Slow down, you crazy child*
> *and take the phone off the hook and disappear for*
> *awhile*
> *it's all right, you can afford to lose a day or two*
> *When will you realize....*
> *Vienna waits for you?*

Slow down, time could not be going any slower. This day is taking so long to get through; I just want tomorrow. I'm not crazy today; I'm not on medicine today. I can't even reach my phone to take it off the hook. Disappear? If only. I want to disappear, I want to go away. It's not all right, Billy, it really hurts. Lose a day or two? Try a month or two. There are two places that I would kill to be in right now; the UCLA Pain Management Clinic or – yes – Vienna. Maybe the UCLA Clinic is my Vienna... Maybe that's my way to peace. Vienna is my life without pain.

Chapter Sixteen

When I woke up my mom was still asleep on top of me. The TV was off, which was odd and my dad was sitting on the edge of the bed, staring off into space.

"Dad?"

He turned, "Yeah?"

"What are you doing?" I asked.

He was thinking and looked very sad.

"Dad, you're scaring me."

"Don't be scared," he said avoiding eye contact.

I sat up, forgetting that my mom was asleep on me. Her head plopped down onto the bed and she immediately opened her eyes. "Sorry, mom," I said. She groaned and rubbed her eyes.

"I just got a phone call..." He stopped like he was being tortured. My heart was racing, *what's going on?* "It was from UCLA." *Reminding us of our appointment?* "Your appointment has been moved back."

My eyes started to tear. "What do you mean moved back?"

"The doctor's daughter just went into labor so she had to go out of town."

"Are you kidding me right now?"

He put his head down. "No."

"So what does that mean?" my mom asked. There were tears in her eyes, too.

"Our appointment will be rescheduled when she gets back."

"Which is when?" I whined.

"They don't know."

That's it. My one hope – gone for an unknown amount of time. That's it, what am I supposed to do now? Who knows when I'll get help?

That was the saddest night of my life at the time. I had never been so down and I barely slept at all.

I pretended to sleep though, because I didn't want to talk to anyone. I hid under my blanket; *because if I can't see them, they can't see me.*

But maybe that's the problem. Maybe the fact that I'm hiding is why I'm not getting help. Maybe the fact that nobody can see me is why I am suffering. If I got out from under the blankets, if I revealed myself, would the pain go away?

I feel more protected while hiding under this blanket, but is that a good thing or a bad thing? Would being vulnerable get me more help?

Who even knows I'm here? Who even cares that I'm here?

How much more vulnerable could I possibly get?

I didn't get out of bed all morning. I didn't even turn on the TV, I just laid there in silence. *Is time even moving?*

Why does it even matter if time moves? I'm not going anywhere. Why should time go somewhere when I can't.

I want to grab onto time and hold it with me. I want to preserve my youth and not let it slip through my fingers.

I'm going nowhere.

"Georgia," I heard the door open. "Georgia."

I pretended to wake up. My dad's friend Jaron was in the doorway dressed in his usual sweatsuit.

"What are you doing here?"

"I'm going to lunch with your dad and I wanted to invite you."

"I'm really not doing well today, Jaron, but thanks."

"Come on, just come out with us," he pleaded. "When was the last time you got out of the house?"

I thought about it. It had been a couple of days. "Do I get to pick where we go?"

"So how's everything going?" Jaron asked after the waiter took our order. I'd picked Robbie Mac's for my favorite pizza.

"Horrible," I said looking at my dad across the table. He looked just as beaten down as I probably did.

"I heard about today. I'm sorry."

"Yeah, me too."

"How are your friends doing?"

"Not well." He always had so many questions.

"How are the boys doing?"

"What boys?" I asked sarcastically.

"Oh come on," he said jokingly. "The boys have to be all over a girl like you."

"Yeah, right." *Stop lying to me.*

"When they wise up, trust me, your dad over here is going to have to get a shotgun."

No boy could ever like me; I don't even like me.

It hurts to know that. It hurts to feel this unattractive. Aren't these the years that I'm supposed to be feeling hot and flirting with guys?

I want to feel wanted; I want to have a companion. Will that ever happen for me? Will I be reduced to crutches and a bed for the rest of my life? Who would want a future with someone who has no future?

"So, your birthday is coming up," my dad started. "What do you want for your birthday?"

You can't buy what I want in a store. "I really don't care."

"There's got to be something," he insisted.

You can't give me what I want, I already told you. "Dad, I really don't have anything in mind."

He smiled. "How about an iPhone?"

My heart skipped a beat. "Are you serious?" *An iPhone?*

"Yes." He was loving how excited I was. "Would that be a good birthday present?"

"That would be amazing." I was glowing. "But my birthday's over a month away."

"That's the other good part. Would you be okay with getting your birthday present a little early this year?"

Is this a joke? "I think I could deal with that."

"Well, when you get a chance you can go on the internet and order it."

"Thanks, dad!"

"Mom, it's really bad," I whined grabbing my leg.

"Do you want me to massage it?" she offered.

"No, that won't help."

"But today's your appointment with Dr. Nineteen. We need to leave in less than an hour."

"Are you coming with Dad and me?"

"Yeah, I can make this one." That made me smile.

My regular physician, Dr. Eight, was concerned when she heard that my pain appointment had been cancelled and that I was getting worse. She suggested a colleague who often worked with kids in pain.

Dr. Nineteen was a psychiatrist. *Am I crazy?* He was an older gentleman with an office in Santa Monica. It was a corner room, so two of the walls were all windows. It was cool because you could see so much and it felt so open and friendly.

He gave me a huge packet to fill out with tons of questions and diagrams. I had to put an "X" on the areas of the body where my pain was and then I had to scale it from one to ten, etc. I answered many questions that were ever so slightly different from the last. One would be, *"Do you feel depressed when you are in pain?"* The next might be something like, *"Do you feel close to depressed when you are in pain?"*

I worked through that packet and answered everything in detail. I wrote how many hours a night I slept and how much TV I watched. Some of the questions seemed pointless, but they had to be there for some reason so I just went with it. *Dr. Nineteen, be my hero.*

He asked my parents questions, too, and we answered them all. He watched me and listened until the sun went down and it was completely dark outside of the big glass windows.

He gave me prescriptions for intense medications. They were adult anti-depressants which was not a good thing to hear. My parents and I had to sign releases since some of the medications were not FDA approved for a person my age.

Is something this wrong with me?

After just one week of waiting I was beyond desperate. I'd thought I was desperate before, but not knowing when I would be able to see the doctor at UCLA brought me to a new low. *When is this going to end?*

I was pushing all the sand out of my bed thinking about what a mess I was. *Only I would go through this many stress balls.* I always needed a stress ball by my side, especially during a panic attack. I would squeeze it and take all my anger out on it; *that's what they're made for.* But I would always manage to destroy them. Again and again.

My dad kept asking, "How do you pop a stress ball?"

I don't know; they're made to be squeezed! *That's all I did – squeeze, squeeze, squeeze, and squeeze again.*

My sister had a soccer tournament on a beautiful Saturday. My dad took her to the game while my mom babysat me. I felt awful keeping my mom at home because she absolutely loved watching us play sports. *I ruin everything.*

My mom and I just sat in her room all day playing Monopoly. I was having a bit of pain, but I fought through it by focusing on kicking my mom's butt.

"George? Georgia?!"

"Huh?" I groaned opening my eyes. My mom was crouched over me with an extremely worried look on her face. *I have never seen this expression before.* "What happened?"

"Nothing honey," she stroked my hair. "You passed out."

"Then why are you looking at me like that?" I sat up and looked at her eye to eye.

"Am I supposed to get used to seeing my baby pass out?"

"I guess not."

A full game of Monopoly takes a while. It was late afternoon by the time I beat my mom. It was close for a while and I was worried, but I pulled through with my little shoe game piece.

"Do you wanna play again?" I asked.

"No, maybe later," she said, picking up all the pieces and putting them in the box.

"I'm pretty hungry."

"Okay, me too. What do you wa...."

"Close the door."

"Close the door, Veronica!"

Stop yelling!

I opened my eyes to my mom crying and my dad watching me like I was bewitched or something.

"What's going on?" I asked.

My dad raised an eyebrow. "How do you feel right now?"

"I feel like usual, why?"

He glanced at my mom and then explained, "When you passed out, you kind of shook."

"What do you mean?"

"Your mom said you did this earlier today. When you passed out, your whole body shook."

"You mean like a seizure?" It wasn't making any sense.

"Yes, like a seizure."

I had only seen someone have a seizure once in my life and it just happened to be that year. On the last day of the semester Ms. Loya wanted a class picture. We all stood along the wall of the room. When she counted to three and clicked the camera to take the picture, two things happened; the flash went off and Dylan went down.

I can still hear the sound of Dylan flapping on the floor so clearly. I hear girls screaming and everyone running around. I hear the paramedics come and I hear him being carted away. That was a horrible thing to witness. Someone my age going through that was hard to watch.

But that's not me, I don't have seizures. "How is that possible?"

"We don't know," my dad said.

I started to cry, "What's happening?"

"George, George," my mom held me. "Don't have a panic attack. Stay here with us."

My dad spent the rest of the day calling every doctor that he could but it was a Saturday afternoon, so he couldn't really talk to anyone. He left desperate messages and begged doctors to call him back. He even called a family friend in North Carolina who is a therapist, but she couldn't help. *We just want answers.* Another day of waiting, that's all it was.

Finally my pediatrician, Dr. Eight, called him back and they had a long conversation. She said that if it were an epileptic seizure, I would wake up disoriented and not know where I was. That was not the case. She also told us that I would lose control of my bladder, so every time I had a seizure I would urinate; also not the case. She didn't know what was going on and was just as alarmed as we were.

"Do you think you should go to the hospital?" my mom asked when my dad came in the room.

"What do you think?" he asked looking at me.

I was so close to having a panic attack and I was extremely jittery. I shook my head violently and repeatedly whispered, "No, no, no...."

"Are you sure?" he asked.

"Yes, dad! No hospitals, no hospitals!" I was going crazy.

"Why not, honey?" My mom seemed to really want me to go.

"Hospitals don't help. Doctors don't help."

"Oh, but Peaches..." My mom made a disappointed face. "Sometimes they do, Peaches."

"No, no, they don't." She could not change my opinion, no one can.

"I think we should go," my dad added.

"You of all people should know what I'm talking about!" I snapped. *Why was everyone ganging up on me?*

"I do know what you're talking about, but I also know that if we don't get help, and these seizures turn out to be serious, it could be catastrophic. We need someone to look at you." He was pleading with me at this point.

"What?" I said sarcastically. "So we go tonight, Saturday, and a doctor sees me on Monday just to throw his hands up and tell me that he doesn't know? What's that going to accomplish?"

"We have to try."

Chapter Seventeen

"Huston, no 'o,'"
"First name?"
"Georgia."
"Okay, Miss Huston. Please have a seat and we will be with you as soon as possible." She gave me a fake smile. I could tell it was fake. I don't know how, but it was.

I walked over to my dad and imitated her voice. "As soon as possible." I made a face. "As soon as possible."

I was angry. I didn't want to be there, they couldn't help me. *What a waste of time.*

"Let's go, dad. Please," I begged.
"We have to stay."
"You know they aren't going to help." *I have every doctor figured out, I know what they do and how they think.*
"You don't know that. We need to explore all our options; we need help."

We arrived at 6:05 p.m.. At 7:37 I was brought in for the usual meet and greet with someone who typed my symptoms into a computer. Then I was sent out until 9:10 when we were moved into a hall. I was given a bed on wheels. *Get comfortable, who knows how long I'll be here.*

"Hi Georgia, my name is Dr. Twenty." 10:23 p.m..
I shook his hand. "Hi."
"So why are we here today?"
I looked at my dad; *go ahead, give him the story.*
My dad went off on his usual rant, but it was longer this time. Every time he tells someone, it gets longer and longer. *When's my "happily ever after – THE END?" When do I get my perfect ending? – Or does it end like this?*

Dr. Twenty thought to himself for a moment. Then he opened his mouth, "So we don't know if she's having epileptic seizures or not? Correct?"

"We don't think she is, because she knows where she is when she wakes up and she still has control of her body," my dad informed him.

"Okay, then it's probably not epileptic. We can't think of anything that could have triggered it? No bright lights or noises?" He was asking me this time.

"No, not that I know of." *Dr. Twenty, be my hero.*

He turned to my dad. "So tell me what she did again."

"I saw one episode, my wife saw both. She passes out, which has been happening pretty regularly, and she shakes violently."

I tried to picture myself lying on the bed having a seizure. I couldn't see it.

"Were her eyes open, closed, or both?"

"Closed."

He thought to himself again. "What doctor are you going to currently?" Dr. Twenty asked.

"Several. And we had an appointment with someone at the UCLA Pain Management Clinic last Monday, but she suddenly had to go out of town. Our appointment was postponed, but we don't know until when."

Dr. Twenty looked pleased. "Dr. Twenty-one?"

"Yeah."

"At this point I think going to her is the best thing that you can do."

"She can really help?" my dad asked, smiling.

"If anyone is going to help you with this pain, it's Dr. Twenty-one." *Yeah, I've never heard that one before. Every doctor's great, every doctor's amazing. I know the truth, I have this all figured out. No one can help me.*

"So does this mean you can't help me?" I asked him snottily.

"I'm sorry." *He didn't seem sorry.* "My advice, just wait until you can see Dr. Twenty-one."

Cool.

Home empty handed. I'm so sick of taking hit after hit of bad news. I want my "happily ever after."

The second I walked through the door my Mom came and hugged me.

"Mom, you didn't have to wait up," I said with her hair in my mouth.

"Yes, I did. What'd the doctor say?" she asked eagerly.

"What do you think?" I said rudely and walked away.

"That's not exactly what he said," my dad interrupted. *How could he be taking his side?!*

"Oh yeah?" I turned. "Then what'd he say? He can't help me! There's nothing else to it."

"He did say that, but he also strongly believes that Dr. Twenty-one can help us. He really made a big deal about her."

My mom smiled. "Oh that's great, honey!"

"No it's not!" I snapped. "Have you guys not caught on yet? Doctors don't care and everything they do is to save their egos!"

"Georgia," my mom whispered, "your sister's sleeping."

"Whatever," I said storming out of the room. "All he did was make me someone else's problem."

I went in my room and collapsed into my own bed for the first time in a while. I wasn't in the mood to go into their room and have to talk to them; *my room, my space.*

It was weird being back in my room. It was really messy, but I really didn't care. It had turned into the family storage unit since I wasn't using it anymore.

I looked around at all the pictures on my walls; me smiling with friends, laughing with friends. I saw my trophies and medals on the bookshelf; my glory days. I saw all my cute, stylish, form-fitting clothes hanging in the closet; back when I had self-confidence and wasn't reduced to a sweatpants, t-shirt combo – back when I was normal.

I told them this would happen. I told them this ER visit would be a waste of time.

I heard my mom open my door and peek in, but I pretended to be asleep.

I fell asleep that night angry; angry at Dr. Twenty, angry at the system, and angry at myself.

Why am I on the floor? Why does my head hurt?

I slowly got up and crawled back through the darkness into my bed and under the covers.

"Peaches," my mom laughed. "What are you doing on the floor?" *Again?*

I opened my eyes and groaned; my head really hurt.

"Wait," my mom realized what had happened. "Did you have a seizure and fall off the bed?!"

"How would I know?" I was grouchy.

"Jimmy!" my mom called.

My dad ran in. "What?"

"She had a seizure last night and fell off the bed." *Twice, but I wasn't about to tell them that.*

"Oh God."

We took Veronica's mattress off her bed and moved it into my room. We put it right next to mine like a trundle bed, so that if I were to fall off again, I would just fall onto Veronica's mattress. Veronica was moved into my parents' room.

I liked sleeping in my room instead of theirs. I hadn't in a while and it was nice to have alone time with just me. It was nice to not have the TV on, so I could listen to my own thoughts and get reunited with myself again. I missed being me.

I woke up the next morning on Veronica's mattress, but my head still hurt. We decided that I might have hit it on the night stand next to my bed, so my mom covered that with pillows. It was like when Sarah was born and we babyproofed the house by putting pads on every hard corner. I was a baby; I couldn't control anything and I needed to be taken care of.

"Can you play Monopoly with me?" I asked Veronica.

"No, you always win," she complained.

"So," I begged, "it's so much fun to play."

"Yeah, for you."

"Come on, please."

"No."

"Pleaseeee."

"Okay fine, but you owe me."

"Do you want to buy Illinois?" I asked her, hoping with all my might that she wouldn't.

"Yes," she grinned, "yes I do."

"Cool," I said jokingly sarcastic and handed her the red property deed.

She took it and waited for a couple of minutes in silence. "Are you even going to school anymore?"

"Not really."

"You're so lucky. I hate school."

That didn't sound like Veronica. She was a great student in a special accelerated school program.

I hated to ask, but – "Why is that?"

"I never do my homework, projects, or study, so I am doing really badly. And I always get picked up so late and I'm always stressed. Everyone at my school makes me mad because they don't understand."

"Understand what?"

She thought about her words and then said, "What's going on at home."

"No," I said quietly, "what's going on with me."

She didn't say anything.

This isn't just ruining my life, it's ruining hers, too. From her point of view I am the enemy; I'm the one ruining her life.

I'm the one she needs to babysit instead of going out with her friends. I'm the one that everyone pays attention to while she gets forgotten at school. I'm the one who sits in bed while she does my chores. I'm the one who wants company when she really needs to work on her schoolwork. I'm the one making her feel alone. I'm the one messing everything up.

Will I ever recover?

Will she ever recover?

"I don't know, she just fell and started shaking," I heard Veronica explaining to my dad.

I opened my eyes and slowly sat up. A game piece was stuck on my face and even when I took it off, I had the impression on my cheek. I looked down and our game was ruined. Monopoly money was everywhere and all my properties were gone. My perfect little world was gone.

I was so sick of lying in my parents' bed watching TV. I was so drained from doing just nothing. I got up and went into my room. *I need something to do.*

I got a huge piece of paper and put it on the floor. I stared at it with anger and resentment, all I wanted was to disappear into the blank paper and live in a blank world without any complications.

I started to get angrier seeing how simple life could be, just like a plain piece of paper, but how mine wasn't at all. I wanted to change that, I wanted to expose people. I wanted a masterpiece.

Who am I most mad at? Myself. Who besides me? Doctors.

Why am I so mad at doctors? It's their job to help me and they aren't doing it. They pretend like they understand or care or want to help, but they don't; all I get are lies.

Lies are what I hate. Lies are what eat me alive. All I want is the truth, but I can never get that. I want to expose the lies and have everyone know the truth. I was still on a lot of heavy drugs.

I kept staring at the big paper, seeing dark colors emerging. I could see children's sad faces and adults huddled in corners. I could see dying flowers and vacant highways. I could see a collage forming in my mind.

I went on my computer and printed out a handful of black and white pictures off the internet. *The truth is black and white also, it should be easy to tell the difference.*

I googled everything I was feeling at the time; *alone, fear, hesitant, denial, confused, doubt, distrust....*

I printed them out and spread them all around the floor of my room. I cut out the ones that stood out to me and put them in a pile. When I had all my pictures, it was time for the fun stuff.

I went through my art drawer, which is just a bunch of random things that I think I might use one day, and took out colorful pieces of paper. I made a collage of those bright prints and interesting designs on the big blank paper in my room.

Then I put out all the pictures and sorted them in the way I thought looked best. I put the dead flower and the live flower in the upper left corner, and under it a waterfall. Next to the waterfall was a man covering his eyes, and on the other side was a lonely fence along the side of a deserted highway. Above that was a group of small African children lined up and looking very unhappy. Under them was a little ballerina in a tutu and she was covering her face with her arms. Next to her was a girl with her knees drawn up and her face hiding as she huddled in a huge, empty hallway. Then there was an old woman putting her hand to her mouth like she was concentrating on something. Beneath her is a sloppy sketch of harsh lines making a faint outline of a person. There were a lot of people covering their faces, hiding in corners. There was a man screaming and to his right was an empty shed on an empty property.

When I thought that all of the pictures were in the right spots, I started to add little details. I put a couple of colored flower stickers around. On the only girl not hiding her face, I put a cage-like sticker so you could barely see her. I took a "Y" sponge, dipped it in white paint, and dabbed the "Y" in various spots; it ended up smudging in some areas so to others it may seem just like a triangle – it's a "Y;" *like why is this happening to me?*

I typed the word "LIES" in a bold plain text and cut around the letters. I put that word in the only empty spot on the page; the upper right corner. *It still needs something else.*

I painted the bottom of my foot with orange paint and stepped on a random spot on the page; just like the doctors and lies were walking all over me. I was returning the favor and walking back on them.

When I stepped back and saw what I had done I was extremely satisfied. It was like a therapy for me, getting all my feelings out. I saw the layers of color, covered by the black and white photos of sadness; just like my layers of color and happiness had been buried. I saw myself in every single one of those photos.

"Georgia, Jordan's here," my mom called, opening the door with him right behind her.

I pulled my blanket up to my chin and pretended not to be bothered at the fact that my mom didn't give me any warning.

"Hey."

Jordan came in and sat on the bed with me. "Hey, whatsup?"

We hadn't seen each other in a while and it was obvious how awkward we were both feeling. "Not much."

"So you're out of your body cast," he said slowly.

"Yeah, for a couple of weeks now," I answered. "What are you doing here?"

"My mom wanted to bring over a casserole for you guys."

"Well thanks, that's nice. What have you been up to?"

"Just hanging out. How about you?"

"Nothing really."

I wanted to talk it up. I wanted to make it seem like I had an amazing life – but I couldn't. My life sucked. One of my best friends had become a complete stranger to me. All my friends had become strangers to me. Why am I distancing myself from everyone who cares?

A week after our last call from UCLA, we got another call; a good call.

"Georgia," my dad announced, "we have an appointment next week."

"What day?" I asked glowing.

"Monday."

I just have to get through six more days. I can do it.

Chapter Eighteen

"Georgia? What are you doing over here?" my mom asked the next morning.

"Huh?" I was sprawled across the floor of my room right next to the door. "I don't know."

"Did you fall asleep over here?"

"No mom. Why would I fall asleep on the hard wood floor?" I asked sarcastically. My body was aching while I got up.

"Do you think you could have been sleepwalking? Or maybe you were on your way to the bathroom in the middle of the night and just passed out?" She was digging for any logical explanation for why I woke up across the room.

"I don't know, mom. I was asleep."

"But you have to have some idea," she groaned.

"Well, I don't."

After that night my mom covered my whole room with pillows, thick blankets, towels, and bundled up sheets from all over the house. She took stuffed animals, and anything else soft she could find, and covered everything that was hard or sharp because there was no telling what went on in there at night.

It was like when there are crazy people and they don't want them to hurt themselves. They stick them in padded rooms – where the floor and walls are just soft pillows, so there is no way for them to hurt themselves. It's a really sad and depressing feeling to be a danger to yourself.

Why did I wake up across the room? Was I possessed? I had seen that in movies and scary TV shows. Maybe my room was haunted.

I was watching a movie in my parents' room while my mom was at work and my sister was at school. It was just my dad and me at home. I was concentrating on the movie when I blacked out again. I woke up on the floor in the hallway, with my dad standing over me.

"What happened?" he asked.

"I don't know," I answered, rolling over so that I wasn't face down in the carpet.

"Did you pass out while you were walking again?" He was trying to find logic in why I was there and not in bed.

"No, I wasn't going anywhere."

"Maybe you just don't remember, but you were on your way to the bathroom."

"No dad, I wasn't. I was lying in bed watching the movie."

"You obviously weren't, because I heard a thud and you were right here."

"You heard me fall?" I asked.

"Yes, it was pretty loud."

"But I really don't remember getting up."

"You must have."

What's going on?

That night I slept in my parents' room with my mom, and my dad slept in my room. We wanted to see what was going on at night and why I was ending up across the room.

Whenever my mom wants to go to sleep she turns on the National Geographic Channel or the Discovery Channel and puts on boring documentaries. Her logic is that she needs the TV on in the background to fall asleep, but if she puts on something interesting, she would watch it instead of going to sleep. It makes sense and it works.

We had our boring documentary on, but what occasionally happened was my mom actually got into that, too, so she stayed up to watch TV. I, of course, fell asleep – because both history and science bore me, and that's usually what documentaries are about. That was when my mom saw firsthand what was really going on.

She said I had a seizure and then I started sleepwalking. I was in such a deep sleep that she couldn't wake me by calling my name or shaking me. She said I got out of bed like a zombie and walked straight into the closed door. I fell onto the floor and then started shaking until I woke up, confused by how I had gotten there.

Something was taking over me while I slept, and sometimes in the middle of the day, too. It was like I was possessed and my body had been taken over by some sort of evil.

In a way that was what was happening. This mysterious pain was my evil that was taking over and I had no control over it. It was taking me to strange places, emotionally and physically. Being taken away by my pain was just as scary and ominous as if I was possessed by a ghost or a demon. I felt screwed either way.

After that night, my parents decided it was time to change around the sleeping arrangements. Again. They moved the couch in front of the fireplace so that I wouldn't hurt myself there. They put my mattress and Veronica's mattress on the floor in the living room, next to each other, so that it made one huge bed. They made a perimeter of pillows and blankets, just like in my room, and then I was set.

I would sleep on the floor in the living room with one parent, while the other one slept in their bed with Veronica. They would alternate nights. I felt like such a burden, and the reality was that I was a burden. I was making life so much harder than it had to be for everyone.

I could feel the happiness drained from the household and it was all my fault. There was no small talk anymore, and there were no smiles. Everything revolved around me, and since depressing things were happening to me, everyone was always in a depressed mood. Visitors would pop in every once and a while and bring a new smiling face, but eventually they would go and the four of us were left alone again.

I couldn't go out. When I went out there was danger everywhere. I could fall and hit my head on the sidewalk again, or I could fall in a restaurant and hit my head on the table. I was a walking hazard and things were only getting worse.

I was imprisoned in my home, and so was my family. They had to watch me every second of every day, because now that I had started unconsciously walking, there was no telling what could happen. Their lives became whatever my life was, and my life was crap.

Chapter Nineteen

"Okay, Peaches. I'm ready," my mom said closing the bathroom door. Things had gotten so bad that I couldn't even take a shower by myself. I needed my mom in there with me to make sure I didn't pass out and hit my head on the tile or drown.

Showers had always been my "me time." I know they are for other people, too, but they really were something that I would look forward to. Before all this, I would sit there and close my eyes, letting my pores soak in the steam. I would sit right under the faucet and watch the water droplets race down the tile walls. Ever since I was a little kid I would guess which one would get there first and then watch as they ate up smaller ones in their path to the bottom, sometimes slowing down and sometimes speeding up.

I would sit there with the water running down my face and think about everything. I would close my eyes and ears so that my mind was blank. I would try to lose myself with water and let my mind wander.

I would reflect on my day and think about my dreams. The shower was the place that I would go to solve problems. For some reason, things that didn't make sense in the real world always fit together like a puzzle in the shower. It was my alone time that I treasured and something that I never thought in a million years would or could be taken away from me.

But like everything else, my shower time, my happy time, had been taken away. I couldn't even do something as private as a shower by myself anymore. I know it was just my mom taking it with me, I wasn't embarrassed at all. It was the principle behind that and how one of the simplest things that everyone on the planet, even little kids, did on a daily basis was out of my reach. Everything was out of my reach.

"Here are your pills," my dad handed me a couple of different colored pills and a cup of water.

"Which ones are these?" I asked, swallowing them without the water.

I was becoming quite the expert.

"These are the pain killers."

"But they don't even work."

"I know, but these are the strongest pain killers that a fourteen-year-old girl can take."

"They make me so loopy, dad."

"I know and I'm sorry. I have to go to a lunch meeting. Are you going to be okay?"

"Yeah, I'll just watch a movie or something."

"Call me if you need anything."

I hated the way I felt after taking the medication. I was on hard-core drugs so they were having hard-core effects on me. *What was that noise? Did the gate just open?*

My mind would go everywhere when these drugs were in my system. I would get totally buzzed. Some people spend lots of money to get buzzed and they think it's the best thing ever. *Who opened the front door?* It wasn't for me; it scared the hell out of me. *Is someone else home?*

I hated feeling out of control and that's exactly what the medications made me feel like; they didn't even give me pain relief so it was a lose-lose.

"Veronica?" No answer. *Did mom come home from work early?* "Mom?"

Who is in the kitchen?

My heart sank; *someone broke into the house.*

I reached over and grabbed my crutches; it had gotten to the point where I couldn't walk without them. I started to get up and then thought against it. *What if they hurt me?*

I thought about my friend who once told me about people breaking into his house – but they didn't hurt him because he pretended to be asleep. I quickly closed my eyes and tried to look asleep, but my breathing was way too fast; a dead giveaway. *Who's washing the pots and pans? Get out of my kitchen.*

What if they hurt my dogs? I can't leave my babies out there with this robber.

I picked up my phone and dialed 9-1 so if the robber tried to hurt me, all I had to do was press "1" to get help. I picked up a crutch to defend myself with. I got the flashlight from under my parents' bed because it was big and really heavy. I could use it to hit the intruder.

The first time I got up I fell back down. *Shhh! Don't give him a warning, don't let him know that anyone's home.* I was so dizzy that I just stopped for a second; I couldn't tell up from down. *What if he takes my computer? I just downloaded a new CD onto it.*

My heart was beating out of my chest, more so than even a panic attack. I literally feared for my life as I slowly opened the door and walked out into the dimly lit hallway.

I heard a noise in the laundry room; *he heard me, he's hiding.*

I walked through the living room, but I couldn't get past the dining room; I was too scared. I couldn't breathe, yet I was breathing so heavily and I was seeing spots everywhere.

I turned around and hopped as hastily and as quietly as I could back into the safety of my parents' room. There were no locks on the doors so I leaned my crutches on both of the doors. *Good luck getting in now.*

I dove onto the bed and covered myself with blankets; *if I can't see him, he can't see me.*

"Get out of my house!" I yelled. *Shhh! Don't let him know you're in here.*

I didn't know what to do, so I called my dad.

"Hello?"

"Dad," I whispered, "there's someone in the house."

"What are you talking about," his voice immediately sounded alarmed.

"Someone broke into the house," I whispered even more quietly.

"How do you know?"

"I can hear them in the kitchen." I jumped as I heard another door slam shut.

"You can hear someone in the kitchen?" He was breathing faster than before.

"Yes dad," I cried quietly. "Please help me, I'm scared."

"Okay, let me think," he paused.

"Should I call 911?"

"No, I'm going to call you right back."

What?!

"Everything's going to be okay."

Did he even believe me?

"Hello?" I answered.

"Phyllis is going to come over," he informed me. "Call me when she gets there."

"When will she be here?"

"She's leaving work right now."

I turned up the volume on the TV really loud. I didn't want to hear the sounds anymore. I knew he was out there; *why was he torturing me?*

Knock, knock.

Oh my God, he's here.

"Georgia?"

Phyllis?! "Yes, I'm in here," I cried out to her.

She opened the door and I had never been so happy to see her before in my life. Don't get me wrong, she wasn't exactly a bodyguard, but she did make me feel safer.

"I heard you needed some company," she smiled, sitting on the bed.

"I need to call my dad and tell him you're here," I said, dialing. "Hey, she's here… yeah, okay. Here she is."

"Hello? Yeah, everything's fine. I checked everywhere… Okay, see you soon. Bye," she handed me back the phone.

No one turned out to be in the house, but I completely believed that there was. That was the first real demonstration of what the drugs did to me. It scared all of us.

I was lying in bed with three days left before my appointment with Dr. Twenty-one, stressing out. *What if the appointment gets canceled again?* There was no way I could deal with another punch like that.

I missed my old life; I missed my friends. My parents were always trying to have me invite my friends over, but honestly I was too embarrassed. I didn't want anyone to see me like this, but that night I just decided to take Solene and Raquel up on their offer. I invited them over.

The next day I was watching TV on the floor of my living room, bored out of my mind. I wasn't in the mood to draw and I wasn't in the mood to play Monopoly. I wanted do anything but be where I was at the moment. I was all alone with my thoughts, and my thoughts sucked. I was left to just be with myself, but I didn't even like myself anymore, so even that wasn't a good thing.

I hated myself. I hated myself because my life was going so great before I started making up this pain. *Am I making it up? It doesn't feel like I am, but I have to be at this point, don't I? But if I am making it up, why can't I just stop it already? I must be crazy. That's the only way.*

"Oh no, oh no," my dad was saying over and over again under his breath.

I opened my eyes and I was on the floor in the dining room with my dad standing over me again. When I sat up, my dad looked like he had seen a ghost.

"Are you okay?" he asked me.

"Yeah," I said, but once I sat up, it hit me. I got so dizzy and almost fell again. My head and right knee were killing me. "No," I said grimacing and lying back down.

"What's wrong?" he asked sitting down next to me.

"My head and knee really hurt," I said grabbing my head. "My head especially."

"Are you seeing okay?"

"Kind of," I said, "there's some stuff that's fuzzy."

"Can you stand up?"

"Yeah, but what happened?"

"I came in here and you were shaking. Then you got up and just bolted into the dining room. You tripped over a chair and hit your head on the wall. Then you fell back and started seizing again."

"It really hurts," I whined, "What do you mean I bolted?"

"You were in a full-on sprint. You just shot up and blindly ran into the chair."

Ran? What was I running to?

I laid back down, scared out of my mind. *What was going to happen next?* I didn't know if I was going to pass out again; *and if I did where would I wake up?* I was scared out of my mind because now, not only was I losing consciousness, but I was doing things while I was unconscious; things that could seriously hurt me.

I wanted to get out of my body, to somewhere I had control and where I felt safe. I managed to feel scared and vulnerable lying on a mattress on a floor where nothing could possibly hurt me – except for myself.

I watched TV for a couple of hours, fell asleep, and surprisingly when I woke up I was in the same place. That made me feel confident and happy, so I decided I was going to go in my room and get my sketchbook to draw. I felt enlightened and inspired; I woke up right where I fell asleep. *I'm getting better!* When I was low – almost every second of every day – something as little as that can feel so life-changing that I became delusional.

I got up and started rummaging through my closet for my sketchbook. When I found it, I just stood there flipping through the pages and looking at my recent drawings. There were some I didn't even remember doing since they were either created while I was on heavy drugs or during a panic attack, when I usually don't remember anything.

I was seeing some of these for the first time and some I liked, some I didn't. Some I thought were beautiful, and honestly some of them scared me. A few made me happy, like my drawings of flowers and my mom. Others made me sad, like the hands of claws or the sad, empty faces. I had a picture for almost every emotion because I was constantly feeling almost every emotion. My life was a roller coaster of emotions that had spiraled out of control and fallen off the tracks. Right now I was falling off the roller coaster and I had no idea what would happen when I hit the ground.

I woke up on the hardwood floor in my room. First I felt my usual throbbing pain in my lower back and head where I must've hit it. Then I opened my eyes and looked up at my ceiling fan, spinning like nothing had happened. Everything in my room looked normal and untouched, yet I was on the floor scared out of my mind.

I tried to get up, but to my absolute horror I could not move a muscle. I couldn't move my fingers, turn my neck, or lift a leg. *Am I paralyzed?!* I literally could not move. *Did I fall and snap my spine?!*

That idea, believe it or not, was not that farfetched. While I was lying there, helpless on the ground, I kept thinking about one of my parents' old friends. She had recently been doing something to her house on a ladder and fell. When she hit the ground she was paralyzed and had to lie there on her driveway until someone eventually found her. That scenario kept running through my head.

I knew it was only a matter of time until my dad came in and found me there paralyzed, but it felt like forever. I tried to make noises to get his attention, but at first only whispers were coming out. I felt like the girl from "Titanic" when she can't get anyone's attention, so they can't save her. *I need a whistle right now, like her.*

I thought about crawling to the chair in my room because if I knocked it over, it would make a loud noise and my dad would come in – but I could not even extend my arm to push it. I was stuck.

I had nothing to do besides think. I thought about all the things that I had always hoped to do, but now that I was paralyzed, I couldn't ever do. I thought about the things that I would never be able to do again. I would never be able to see Golden Hour on a walk with my mom, or walk up the stairs at my school.

But you know that when the truth is told....
That you can get what you want or you can just get old
You're gonna kick off before you even
Get halfway through
When will you realize, Vienna waits for you?

The truth is hardly ever told; that's why it is so cherished. Everyone wants the truth so badly, but society is constantly manipulating it and using it against us. I can't get what I want and I probably won't even have a chance to get old. I am wasting away and there is nothing anyone can do about it. I'm going to "kick off." I'm going to die. I'm going to die before I even get halfway through. A fourteen-year-old should never have to think that they are going to die, but I don't think — I know. I guess Vienna is not somewhere that I will ever reach in my life; maybe it's what happens to me when I die — or maybe it's something that I will never see.

Chapter Twenty

It's such a strange feeling to not be able to move at all; *maybe I already am dead. Maybe this is the process of death. Maybe this is my redemption period. Some people say that they died and they had a choice; whether to proceed to the afterlife, and whatever that has to offer, or to go back to Earth and live their lives. Am I ready to die?*

I reflected on my life while I was lying there staring up at my ceiling fan. I thought about playing sports and the joy I got out of playing with a team. I thought about how far I had gone and how many trophies I'd earned in multiple sports. I thought about how I was the only one out of all my middle school friends to get into Notre Dame and what an accomplishment that was. I thought about where my funeral would be.

I thought about all the art that I did that I never showed anybody. I thought about how I was going to die before my grandparents and how it is not supposed to be like this. I thought about how rude and unappreciative I was the last time I spoke to my sister. I thought about how dismissive I was when my mom asked me how my day was yesterday. I thought about all the questions that my dad had fought so hard to find answers for, that will always be unanswered. I wasn't ready to die.

I heard my dad get out of his chair in the room just across the wall. *Please open the door to come in my room.*

"Dad," I called out pretty loudly, "dad, dad, dad." After a couple of yells my door opened.

"What happened?" he asked crouching down next to me.

"I can't move," I whispered. It hurt to even talk.

"What do you mean you can't move?" He started freaking out.

"I can't move," I repeated painfully.

"What happened?!"

"I don't know."

"How long have you been here?"

"I don't know."

"Are you in pain?"

"Yes."

"I'm going to call 911 again."

"No, no." That was the last thing I wanted.

"Okay, what do you want me to do?" he asked helplessly.

"I don't know."

"Just tell me what you want me to do," he pleaded.

"Just leave me here."

"Hang on," and he left. He brought the phone into the room and started calling doctors, but of course it takes forever to talk to a doctor directly, in person or over the phone.

I just laid there and eventually, after what seemed like forever, but was really a little over an hour, I started to get feeling back in my body. It started in my hands and arms, then my neck and back, and at last I could feel my legs. My dad and I were so relieved and confused when I could finally stand up. *What happened?*

Another long day went by of me being alone and waking up in random places with random bruises. *Just admit me to an institution already.*

What if I'm a witch? What if this is the Salem witch trials all over again? Am I going to be burned at the stake?

I had been to Salem, and I had learned about that time period throughout my whole life. Everyone blames those girls for ruining the town and being responsible for many innocent people's deaths. *What if it wasn't their fault? What if I am getting the story from their perspective?* There were many similarities between my current state and what they supposedly went through.

There are at least two sides to every story and what if theirs is just as genuine as the rest? What if they were just as scared as the community? I knew that was not the case and that they were being mischiefs; *but what if?*

If I'd lived in that time period – suffering like this – I would have definitely been accused of being involved with witchcraft.

I woke up and felt extremely nervous. It was two days until my appointment with Dr. Twenty-one, but this was the day Solene and Raquel were coming over. *Were they still going to like me?*

My mom kept reminding me of my experience with Ella and how it went great, but it didn't help. I was worse now than I had been when Ella saw me, and I was closer with Ella than I was with these girls. *Are they going to tell everyone at school what I'm like now — weak and pathetic?*

When they walked through the front door and saw me lying on the floor in the living room, I think they were both a little shocked. Solene was holding a huge "Get Well" balloon that made me smile.

It wasn't awkward at all. They sat on the mattresses with me and we talked. I asked how school was and they asked how I was. After a while I invited them to play Monopoly and they were fine with that.

Just as we were setting up the board, my uncle Steve and Sarah surprised me by coming over. Sarah marched in carrying a pink bunny rabbit stuffed animal that was bigger than she was. She proudly handed it to me. They played Monopoly with us.

We were all having fun, joking around and buying properties, when I lost consciousness – the last thing I wanted to do in front of them.

When I woke up everyone was staring at me, including my mom who I guessed they had called in. I looked at Solene and Raquel's shocked faces and was so embarrassed. *Had I just passed out or had I seized also?* No one said anything. I didn't know what to do.

"Whose turn is it?" I asked, collecting my money from next to me where I must've dropped it. I pretended like nothing happened, like I didn't know why they were looking at me so strangely. All I wanted them to do was go home, so I could sink back into my hole where no one else could judge me.

When I went to bed that night I was still embarrassed from what had happened. *How could I have done that in front of them? Now they are never going to want to be my friends again — not that it matters anyway, because I don't even go to school anymore.*

"Here are your pills." My dad handed me a fistful and my water.
"Thanks." I took them.
"Do you want anything to eat?"
"Yeah, I'm hungry."
"What do you want?"
"Pasta with red sauce?"
"Okay," he opened the door to walk out.
"Wait, can you ask Veronica to come in please?"

"Hey George," she popped into the room. "Whatsup?"

"Can you come in," I asked pathetically, "and stay with me a little?"

"I have a school project I really have to do."

"Please? You can do it in here."

"Fine."

Even if we weren't talking, it still felt better to have someone in the room with me. I was always so lonely in that room.

"Can we watch that movie you saw with Ella?" she asked me.

"'Fool's Gold'?"

"Yeah."

"What about your school project?" I smiled.

She smiled back, "I'm taking a break."

We'd just started the movie when my dad came in with my pasta.

"Thanks, dad."

"You're welcome. Do you want some, Veronica?"

"No thank you," she answered.

"Will you guys be okay if I step out for a meeting?"

"Yeah," we both said, eyes glued to the TV.

"Call me if you need anything," he said closing the door.

"Do you think that actor's cute?" Veronica asked me.

"Which one?"

"The one in the yellow."

"He has a good body, but he's not cute."

"I think he's cute."

"Yous think everybody's cute."

"No, I don't."

"But yous don't dink handsome people are cute which is finny," I laffed.

"What are you talking about?"

"Nuffing," I made a silly fase ad her.

"What's going on?" She looked concerned. "Why are you talking like that?"

"Like nuffing!" I exklamed.

She started laughing. "Did you just take your medicine?"

"I kan't rember." *I reallie kan't.*

She laughed, "You're going crazy."

"Yous the krazie one."

"Seriously though, can you hear yourself?"

"Nope." *Whut wus that noise?*

"Do you want me to turn off the TV?"

"No! Dont!"

"Okay," she giggled. "Okay, just relax."

"Yous relacks." *Whu is inn the kitchin?*

"What are you thinking right now? I'm really curious."

"I um trying to fegure owt whu is en the howse with us," *that us the trooth.*

Her face dropped. "What are you talking about?"

"Dont you hears hym too?"

"Who? Georgia, who are you talking about?" She was giving me such a serious face.

"Shhh... lissen," I holded up my fingur so she wud be quiet.

"What am I listening for?"

Her eyes and ears were opened as wide as could be as she strained everything she had to hear what I was hearing.

"The mann duing the dishis is bak."

Wee stopped tawking and lissened.

"Oh my God!" All the color was gone from her face; she heard him, too. "What do we do?"

"He's hurd to fined."

"What are you talking about?" She was getting hysterical. "What do we do? There's someone in the house!"

"Nuffing," I sud smileing and thruw my head bak into the pellow.

"Where's your phone?"

She was scrambling around the bed, looking for it under the covers.

"Here it es," I handeded it two her.

She dialed my dad and the second he answered she started whispering, "Dad, there is someone in the house."

"He jusd turned on the sinks," I laffed like a krazie persun.

"Yeah, I heard it, too. Dad, he just turned on the sink... Yeah, I really do hear him, too... Okay, but what do we do?... Do you not understa... Okay, tell them to hurry."

"Whud he saye?"

"He's calling Azmi and Christiana. They are going to come help us."

"I um skared," I sud as it suddenley hit me. *The man is bak.*

"It's okay, George." We held each other until Azmi and Christiana came.

Somehow Veronica had caught my hysteria and she started hearing the same noises, even though she wasn't on the heavy medication. If someone tells you that the planet is square enough times, you'll start thinking that the planet is square.

149

My appointment with Dr. Twenty-one was the next day. I just had to make it through one more night and then I would be all better. *After tomorrow I'm not going to have any pain anymore and my life is going to be back to normal. One more day, then everything will be fine.*

I got dressed in a cute outfit for the first time in a while. I was excited to go out to a place where people would understand what I was going through and where I wasn't a freak. Maybe I would make friends with people in the waiting room who had been going through the same things that I was, and who could actually relate to my experiences. I was on my way to get help.

What does she look like? What medicines is she going to give me? On the way to UCLA I was imagining what meeting Dr. Twenty-one would be like. I had been waiting so long, but she had probably not even heard my name until she came into work that morning and saw her patient list. She was like a celebrity to me and just like celebrities don't know all their fans, she didn't know of me.

While we were driving across the UCLA campus I watched all the students hustling around from class to class. Some were sitting down reading books and some were talking with friends. Some looked happy and some looked like they were having bad days.

I wanted that more than anything. I wanted to be with other people my age that I had similarities with. I wanted to have bad days, because if you have a bad day, that means that you also have good days; otherwise you have nothing to compare it to. Some people ask, "Why are there bad things in the world?" Some answer, "Because if there was no bad in the world, we wouldn't know what good was." I know nobody likes bad things happening, but if they didn't then we wouldn't be able to appreciate the good things.

I had been in such a rut for so long, and I knew I was having all bad days, but honestly I hadn't even thought of it that way. A psychological term for what I was going through is anhedonia, which means that I didn't even feel the ups and downs of my life. I had been living with one bad day after another for so long that it had just become routine for me. I didn't even consider my days bad anymore, because at the time they weren't bad, they were normal. All I wanted was a bad day so that I could know that there had at least been a good one recently. Feeling bad is better than not feeling at all.

We found the building and parked under the big medical center. I had to crutch a far distance from the car to the elevator, but it was worth it; *I'm going to be healed today.* With every step I could feel less pain, *her magic is working already.*

As we went up the elevator my heart was beating fast, from feelings that I hadn't felt in a long, long time; excitement and hope. *This is my last day of pain — I'm finally at the UCLA Pediatric Pain Management Clinic!*

When we got to the proper floor, as soon as you get out of the elevator you see kids, but they weren't really the kids that I was expecting – some were going to other doctors in other clinics.

Half the kids in the waiting room were infants and toddlers. One fourth of them were in wheelchairs and had developmental problems, and then probably a fourth looked like me. There was quite a diversity in there, but gosh was that waiting room packed. There were tons of couches. All the cushions were different colors because the place was very kid friendly, yet it was hard to find an empty seat.

My mom and I sat down while my dad signed me in. I was sitting there – waiting – but also watching. I was looking around the room and observing each person. I saw the bags under the parents' eyes and how incredibly tired they all looked. I saw the kids who were going through the pain and how standoffish they seemed, with their arms crossed and scowls on their faces. I saw the little siblings who were dragged to these appointments and how restless they seemed, all fighting for their parents' attention. It wasn't fair. Everyone in that room looked like they had been stretched as thin as they could possibly be. *Is this not the end for us? Does it get worse?*

No, it couldn't. This is Dr. Twenty-one, she is going to help me. Dr. Twenty-one, be my hero.

It was a pretty long and depressing wait, but I knew it would be worth it. When they finally called my name, one of the nurses took me into a room to get my weight, blood pressure, height, and temperature. Then she walked my parents and me down the hallway to my room. The walls were covered with pictures that patients had drawn. Some had the kids flying in the sky, maybe they felt free now, and some had family pictures with Dr. Twenty-one in the family portrait. All and all, they were hopeful and every single one of them thanked Dr. Twenty-one. *Maybe my art will be up there one day.*

I sat with my parents and waited for Dr. Twenty-one to come in. My mind was wondering what she was going to look like and sound like –

what she was going to be like.

When the door opened my heart nearly leapt out of my chest.

"Hi, I'm Dr. Twenty-one," she said smiling. We all introduced ourselves and my dad told her how much he loved her book on chronic pediatric pain.

"It was incredible how similar the stories in it were to ours," he said.

"Yes, it is. A lot of kids have pain, but not a lot of people necessarily believe them," she nodded. Then she looked at me. "Did you read it?"

Oops. "No, I didn't," I answered, embarrassed.

My dad broke in "We asked her if she wanted to, but she said 'no.' Lynn and I read it though."

"That's fine," she laughed. "It's more for the parents anyway. So Georgia, where is your pain?"

"My right leg and lower back," I said.

"Well," my dad interrupted, "can I walk you through the story?"

There he went, starting from Dr. Two, through Dr. Five the acupuncturist. He told her about Dr. Nine and his many casts, and Dr. Six wanting to inject me with deforming steroids. He talked about the nerve test I had done and waiting all night in hospitals, still coming home empty handed. Maybe this was where the story was going to end, right here at UCLA. Maybe there wouldn't be any more additions to my saga of pain.

Every single person we have ever told this story seems shocked and horrified. They can never believe all the things that we had gone through, but strangely she didn't react. Her facial expression didn't change at all while she was writing notes on what my dad was saying. *Is she not hearing this right? Does he need to repeat things?*

While he was telling the story I passed out, and when I woke up my dad was by my side, but Dr. Twenty-one didn't seem alarmed at all.

He continued his story and when he was done she didn't tell us how horrible it all sounded, or how she was sorry that this happened to us. She didn't look at me sympathetically or have to soak it all in. She took the information that he gave her and just went with it.

"I know Lynn and Jimmy have heard of chronic pain from my book. Have you, Georgia?" she asked looking up from her notes.

"No," I said hesitantly. "Is that what I have?"

"Yes," she said. "Lynn and Jimmy, do you understand what it is?"

"I think so, but I think you should explain it to all of us," my dad said.

"Okay, this is what I think happened. When you touch a hot stove, pain from your hand shoots up to your brain and its pain receptors tell you that your hand hurts."

We all nodded.

"When you remove your hand from the stove, it should stop feeling the pain, right? That's because your pain receptors close when you are not touching the stove anymore." *What does this have to do with anything?*

"When you tore those ligaments in your ankle, it was like touching the stove. Your pain went up the nerves to your brain and told your pain receptors that it hurt. But when you healed – like when you remove your hand from the hot stove – your pain receptors didn't turn off."

"That's why you keep feeling this pain that doesn't show up on an X-ray or MRI, because it is not in the back or the leg. When you tell the doctors that your leg and back hurt, they look at your leg and back, when what they really needed to do in this circumstance is focus on your brain. There is nothing wrong with your leg and back."

What the hell? How is there nothing wrong with my leg and back? How can you tell me that there is nothing going on there? I felt extremely misunderstood and it made me frustrated.

She seemed to know I was confused and paused. "Does that make sense?"

No! "Yes."

My dad asked, "So what do we do now that we know what this is?"

"We have a team here at the clinic," she said, handing us identical printouts. "We all have different specialties, but we all work together to help the patients. This list shows all the different therapies we offer. Each patient can go to as many or as few as we think necessary and then once a week all of the team members meet to discuss the patients and their progress. That way we are all on the same page and can understand all the different aspects of the child."

"Are the therapies done here?" my mom asked.

"No, some are at the therapists' homes and some are at their offices. They are all extremely professional though and are, in my opinion, the best at what they do."

"So which therapies should we do?" my dad asked looking at the list.

Whoa, whoa, whoa, slow down. I'm still confused!

"I have a couple in mind. Tell me what you think," she started. "First, I'm going to suggest physical therapy."

"But we already tried that," my mom interjected.

"Yes, but you did physical therapy for the herniated disc, not for chronic pain," she reminded us.

"Can I do it with Debra? She was my physical therapist," I asked;

maybe there is some good out of this. Maybe I will get to spend more time with Debra.

She thought about it. "You can, but I think it would be best if you did it with our physical therapist so you are working within our team."

"We will go to yours," my dad answered for me. My heart sank and my pain increased.

"I also want you to do Iyengar yoga with Beth. Iyengar yoga is a special type of yoga designed for older people or people with injuries. It's less stressful on the body than other types of yoga. I want you to do something called hypnotherapy with Kathryn. She will help you calm down when you're in pain or feeling overwhelmed. Since you like art so much, and you have already been using it as a form of therapy, we have an amazing art therapist, Esther, who I want you to see. You're going to like this next one, Georgia. We have a great guy, Chris, who does craniosacral massage and he can help you get your body back in balance."

"The last thing I am going to suggest is for you, Lynn and Jimmy, to see a family therapist who should help you deal with everything. How does all that sound?" she asked.

We each wondered about it silently until my dad shrugged, "Whatever you think will work."

"Okay, the list has their names and phone numbers. You can make the appointments at your convenience," she said circling all the names she'd just suggested. "Georgia, when was the last time you went to school?"

"It's probably been a month since I've gone," I answered.

"I have a request," my dad interrupted. "Could you write a letter to the school about why she's been absent? Because it's been so long, they need a letter from a doctor."

"Yes, I will do that," she said, making a note and then looking up at me. "What would you say about going back to school?"

"But I'm passing out and everything," I said.

"I'm not saying go to classes exactly. What about just going for a nutrition break, or eating lunch there? Do you think your school would let that happen?"

"Yeah, they would, but what if I pass out?"

"Everything will be okay. Have you been seeing your friends?"

"No, not really."

"I want you to try to get back to your normal life as much as possible, meaning socializing," she said, "and that means getting back to school, even if it's not for classes."

I did not like that idea at all. I hadn't been to school in so long, I couldn't just pop my head back in for half an hour. I wasn't going to do that. I wasn't going to be asked the same questions over and over again; I just wasn't ready for that.

"I'll think about it," I lied.

"Next, our goal is to take you off all this medication." *Huh?!*

"Why?" I asked.

"We want to get rid of your pain and the medicine is obviously not doing that. We could put you on the heaviest pain killers in the world, but it wouldn't help. The drugs are targeting the wrong thing and fighting the wrong fight." Then she paused to think. "But since these are such strong meds, we cannot just quit taking them. You are going to have to slowly wean yourself off them. Who's in charge of the medication?"

My dad raised his hand.

"Okay, we are going to be cutting the pills back each week. Do you understand?"

He nodded.

"They will still be in her system for a while, but slowly we will get her off of them. All I'm going to add is one pill, a small dose of Lexapro. I want that to eventually be the only pill you are taking besides Singular for your asthma." *Oh my God, slow down lady.*

"We can do that," my dad said.

"Now, Georgia," she said, sternly looking at me, "when you're in pain, what do you do?"

"What do you mean, what do I do?" I was confused.

"What's the first thing you do when you are in pain?"

"I don't know. I guess I go to bed and turn on the TV," I said hesitantly.

She nodded. "Don't do that anymore, okay? When you are in pain, the last thing you need to be doing is giving up and feeling sorry for yourself. You need to continue living your life, even if you're in pain. You need to suck it up and fight through it. Don't let this run your life — you run your life."

Easy for you to say. "Okay," I agreed.

"Now if you could go out in the waiting room, I would like to talk to your parents. Then you and I will talk. Is that okay?"

Like I have a choice. "Sure," and I left.

I walked out to the crowded waiting room and sat down on an empty part of a couch. *Can someone explain to me what just happened?*

I felt so overwhelmed and confused, I had no idea what was going on. I felt like everything was just thrown at me at once and I didn't understand any of it.

I still don't even know what chronic pain is. If there is no physical reason, then I am making it up. She said it was in my brain. That means something's wrong with my brain.

My eyes started to water; *all those doctors were right. All those people that I was mad at because they said they couldn't help me, they were all right. Nobody can help me because there is something wrong with my brain, I'm crazy. I am making up all this pain; my worst nightmare has come true. A doctor just verified that I am making this all up.*

I ruined my life.

Chapter Twenty-one

I sat there thinking about how stupid I was for almost ten minutes before my parents came in. It was my turn. I picked up my crutches and hobbled through the door and down the long hallway. *What now?*

She was waiting for me and smiled when I came in. "Hi Georgia. Have a seat."

I sat down cautiously.

"You've been pretty quiet," she started.

"I always am when I'm at a doctor's office," I said blankly.

"Why is that?"

"Nothing I say helps," I said quickly.

"Do you really feel that way?" She seemed surprised.

"Yes."

"Well I can't speak for all doctors, but for me I know that's not the case. Everything you tell me will help because I am here to help." *Maybe she's not so bad after all.*

"Okay." *But I've heard all this before.* "I have some questions I wanted to ask you without your parents here. Is that okay?"

"Yeah," I braced myself. I knew the questions that were coming.

She sat down so we were at the same eye level. "Is there anything going on at home I should know about?" *No, I'm not being abused or anything.*

"No."

"Have you ever been depressed?"

I had to really think about that one. "I think so."

"Why do you think you have been depressed?"

"Because a lot of doctors have put me on anti-depressants and I am always feeling down and alone. I think my life sucks."

"Have you ever been suicidal or thought about suicide?"

"No, never." *I have already inflicted so much pain and suffering on the people I love, why would I add that? I'm not sure if that's the only reason I haven't considered it, but it's a good one.*

"Do you have a significant other in your life?"

How the hell could I fit a boy into my life right now? How the hell could a boy possibly want to be in my life, or even want to spend time with me?

"No."

"Do you miss your friends?"

Why is she asking about such touchy subjects? Stop! These have nothing to do with it!

"I guess."

"Why don't you see them anymore?"

"I don't know," I said, but I really did know. *Because I'm embarrassed; because I am ashamed.*

"I have been dealing with this kind of pain for a long, long time. We all know what we are doing and we are all going to help you."

"That'd be great."

I didn't believe her. It just didn't make sense. *How were hypnotherapy and art therapy going to help my pain?*

"What did you think?" my dad asked when we got in the car.

"I think she's crazy," I said. *Massages cannot stop my pain, and neither can yoga.*

"Yeah, I've never really experienced an approach like this before," my dad agreed.

"Are we going to do it?" I asked.

"Why wouldn't we?"

"Because these aren't things you do for medical problems. These are things that hippies did for recreational purposes."

"Don't you think you should give it a shot?" my mom asked.

"But none of it makes sense," I argued, frustrated.

"Why do you have this pain?" my dad asked.

"I don't know."

"How are you going to stop it?"

"I don't know."

"Exactly," he said, "she does."

That day I went home even more frustrated and confused than ever before. She wanted us to come back in two weeks so she could see my progress. *What progress? I just keep going downhill.* Nothing I did or said alarmed her in any way – *does she just not care?*

My dad started making my appointments for the various "therapies." I had a physical therapy appointment the next day, which I was not looking forward to. I felt like I was cheating on Debra and I did not want to go to anyone else.

I picked up my pencil and drawing pad and got to work. I felt so sad and frenzied that I just had to get something out.

I drew a huge tear drop that extended off the page. I drew two rainbows running into each other, going in opposite directions. I put a mask over a rainbow floating over waves at the base of the tear, like a stormy ocean.

My life used to be the first rainbow, but then my life changed course, completely altering my path. The mask was covering the new rainbow, the one bringing me on the track of self-destruction, floating a mere couple of inches above the stormy water. I made all that with a gray pencil so everything was dark and depressing looking, *the way life is.*

But what if life isn't always depressing? My life had been pretty good before all of this. *What if it can be good again? What if I can change my path and switch rainbows? What if it's up to me?* I looked at the rainbow with the mask and the rainbow without the mask. *I can choose which rainbow I am on.*

I took a pink marker and drew an outline of a flower on the rainbow without the mask. It was the only piece of color on the whole picture, even the rainbows were a blackish gray. It showed that even in the most dismal circumstances, even if I had nothing to work with, I could still determine my own destiny. There would always be some sort of color in my life; I just had to find it.

"Hi, I'm Diane," she said when we walked into the gym.
"I'm Georgia," I replied. "Nice to meet you."
"You too," she smiled. "What do you say we get to work?"
"Okay."

I followed her as she walked me around the physical therapy area. "Have you ever done physical therapy before?" Diane asked.
"Yeah, a couple of times," I answered.
"Okay, we're going to start here," she said and showed me the exercise that she wanted me to do. It seemed easy enough, but it was hard not being able to use my crutches. It was also the only physical activity that I had done for months and even though it was a pathetic little exercise, I was going through hell to try to get it done. *Am I the same star athlete as before?*

I was feeling pain everywhere, but I was determined to work through it. It was my first time and I wasn't going to let her see me as weak. It got to the point where I was crying from the pain, but I didn't let her see. It was an overwhelming experience that I wasn't up for.

I didn't like physical therapy and decided that I wasn't going to do it anymore. Maybe it was because it was too hard for me or because it wasn't Debra I was doing it with. I had no idea; all I knew was that I didn't want to do it again. *Maybe this stuff isn't going to work for me after all.*

My next appointment was Iyengar yoga, and I had absolutely no idea what to expect. I tried to picture what I would be doing while I was trying to fall asleep the night before. I thought back to when I was little and my mom cut out a magazine article showing and explaining some yoga poses. She decided that she, my sister, and I would get involved with yoga in the back yard. I'll never forget it because all the pictures in the magazine article were of a mother and daughter doing it together.

Veronica ended up quitting pretty early, so it was just my mom and me. We were doing our best to imitate the odd poses that the pictures showed and laughing our asses off when we failed miserably. I remember how weird the names were for the poses and how we made up our own poses based on the names and what we thought they should look like.

How the heck is yoga going to stop my pain? Isn't it just for recreational purposes? I used to be so flexible, but ever since all this happened I have completely lost it; *I probably can't even touch my toes anymore.*

I was watching TV – with my dad snoring on the floor next to me in the living room – wondering where my life had gone. *Now that I know that it's all in my head, why can't I stop it?*

Chapter Twenty-two

The next morning I woke up on the carpet in the hallway. I had managed to get from the bed in the living room to the floor in the hallway without waking anyone up – including myself. *How long have I been here?*

I felt something cold and wet on my arm, but I disregarded it at first. Finally I opened my eyes and saw one of my dogs lying next to me. The cold wet thing was her nose touching me. She was just lying there next to me, as loyal as could be. When she saw me looking at her, she licked me. She was there for me. I didn't know how long she had been there, but she was there for me.

I decided I was just going to lie there with her. *What would be the point of going back to bed anyway? I wouldn't stay there.*

I didn't know what time it was and I didn't care. I could tell it was early, early morning so I moved closer to my dog, making her furry belly my pillow, and drifted back to sleep with the warm feeling of safety. I cuddled with my dog on the floor of the hallway until everyone else woke up.

I was not looking forward to yoga as we drove through the Beverly Glen canyon to Westwood. I had no idea what to expect; *was it going to be like when my mom and I tried to copy the people in the magazine?*

I knew that I could never get my body to do the things that they did, especially not at the moment.

We were driving through a very nice neighborhood; *is her office in a house?* After a few minutes of enjoying the warm sun on my face – that I so rarely got to experience nowadays – we pulled up to a big yellow house. It was two stories and absolutely gorgeous. It had flowers everywhere and was extremely welcoming; *well I guess we're here.*

"What's her name again?" I asked my dad, looking at the intimidatingly perfect house with the perfect lawn.

My dad looked down at a piece of paper and read, "Beth."

"Are we too early?"

"We're fine," he said opening his door and getting out.

I waited until he got my crutches and opened the door for me. I hobbled up the steps and rang the doorbell. On the door there was a little Hindu statue of someone praying and in its hands were fresh flowers.

My mom loves flowers, and she taught me to love them, too. On all our walks during golden hour, if we saw a nice looking flower, she would always stop and smell it. I would get irritated because she was always stopping to smell the flowers instead of walking. I used to think they all smelled the same and that she was just wasting time. After a while, I got her flower sniffing OCD, so now I'm obsessed with flowers, too. Everyone always teases me when I stop and smell a flower, but if it looks nice I can't walk by it. *And what's wrong with that? Doesn't everybody always say that we need to take time to stop and smell the roses?*

The door opened and a very happy looking blonde woman in black opened the door. "Georgia?" she asked.

"Yeah, hi," I answered awkwardly.

"I'm Beth," she smiled and took a step back, "come on in!"

Just as I expected, my dad started to tell our story. I zoned out on what he was saying and looked around at what I could see from the hallway. To my left was a huge empty room with hooks and ropes on the walls and a big wooden structure in the corner. I guessed that it was a room she used for yoga. To my right was a smaller room with a bunch of objects that I was unfamiliar with, but the wall also had hooks and rope. There was a big mirror on the wall and a lot of blankets stacked neatly against it. *Did the rest of her house look this nice and clean?* I could see a big staircase and a shut door that probably led to the rest of the house. There were no lights on, but the many windows in the house made it well-lit.

"That sounds awful," I heard her say sympathetically; *time to tune back in, George.* "I'm so sorry you had to go through all that."

"Did I miss anything?" my dad asked me as a joke. I had absolutely no idea, but I shook my head anyway.

"Okay, if you're ready, Georgia, we will get to work. Are you going to be staying?" she asked my dad.

"No, when should I come back?"

"In about an hour." And he was gone.

"So," she turned to me smiling, "as you can tell these are my yoga studios."

"They're really nice," I laughed, "they weren't exactly what I was expecting."

"What were you expecting?" She seemed amused.

"I don't know, doing it in your living room or something. I never imagined such a big operation in your house."

She laughed, "Well, that big room is where I do group lessons, but since it's just us, we're going to be working in here." She brought me into the room with the mirror and all the weird objects. "Have you ever tried yoga?"

"Not really. I just fooled around a few times with my mom."

"I'm sure you'll catch on quickly since you're so athletic."

I couldn't understand or remember ninety percent of the poses that we did that day because most of the names weren't even in English. But the poses didn't have to be in English for them to speak to me.

The human body is pretty much the same for everyone, so it didn't matter that a man in India named B.K.S. Iyengar created it. It spoke to me personally. When I was in child's pose, I could feel every vertebra in my back getting the exact same comfort and stretch at the same time. When I was in triangle pose I could sense that even though my center of gravity had completely shifted, I was more balanced than before. I could feel the ache in the back of my legs while doing downward facing dog. It was an ache that I hadn't felt in a while; it was the ache of being active.

Iyengar yoga is different from other types of yoga because of its unique use of props such as bolsters, blankets, straps, etc. It is used as therapy for older people or people with injuries, which was perfect for me. *It's pretty much yoga for the incapable.*

When my dad picked me up an hour later I found it hard to explain the way yoga made me feel. It felt like I wasn't in my body anymore; it felt peaceful. I did things with my body that day that I never thought I could do, even before all of this. I did stretches with weird names that didn't make sense and held positions for lengths of time that I couldn't believe. It was like it wasn't me anymore.

While I was there I didn't think about school or whether I would have to retake ninth grade or not. I didn't try to figure out what my friends think of me. I wasn't worried about the pain or wondering when my next panic attack was going to be. I was calm and serene; for the first time in months I was genuinely happy.

Maybe this is going to work after all.

When I got home I was sore, but it was a good sore. It was the kind of sore that lets you know that you're working muscles again. It made me feel accomplished; *I finally actually did something!*

I was bored and so sick of TV at this point. I wanted something new; I wanted a challenge. I was feeling so great since yoga and I figured that the best way to express that would be through my art. I wanted to preserve how hopeful I was feeling.

I had been drawing so much lately I decided I wanted to paint. I was never good at painting, but I think that's why I wanted to paint. For me, drawing is such a controlled medium, and that's not what I was in the mood for. When I drew I felt pressure to make it perfect, so every little line was exact. That's not what I wanted right now.

I wanted to express myself in a different way. I wanted to make my mark on paper without planning it out ahead of time, or thinking too far into it; I just wanted to do it. I didn't want a precise drawing with textbook proportions; I wanted a piece of art. I knew I might not like it, because I never liked my paintings, but I didn't care. I decided that for the first time, and it didn't even matter if I never did it like this again, I was going to just go with it and see what happened.

I looked through my art drawer and noticed that I only had white, black, and orange paint; *whatever, just go with it.* I got a pretty big piece of paper and laid it down. I stared at the paper and then back at my paints; *no, don't think – just do it.* I picked up my paintbrush and put it in the black paint first.

I put my paintbrush down and made a pretty big oval with it in the upper right hand corner; *it looks like it should be a face.* I drew an outline of the mouth, nose, eyebrows, and eyes. I stopped before coloring in the eyes; *it looks like a mask.* I kept it like that. I took the orange paint and drew a few thick lines coming out of the mask like sunshine out of the sun. It was looking good so I just did that on the whole page. Then I took the black and white and made a big squiggle on the left side of the page, just to balance it out; that side was looking too empty.

I took a step back. It had only taken about five minutes to do this; *if that's not just going with it then I don't know what is.* I looked at my boring painted face, but surprisingly I wasn't disappointed. I knew it didn't make sense, but while I didn't like it, I was happy with it.

I studied it, trying to find out what it meant. I wanted to know why each line came out of me the way it did. The crude, empty white mask was me; or at least what I felt like. I knew I was hiding but, like before, my mind-set was that if I stayed hidden, not as many bad things could find me. It was like when I hid under blankets because even that thin layer of fabric could protect me. It could protect me because it could hide me. That's what my mask was doing at the time. I didn't mean to be wearing a mask, but I knew I was.

Is the orange shooting into the mask, or away from it? To me, the orange represented hope and a new life. The color orange is said to embody determination and success. *So maybe the orange rays aren't shooting out of me, the mask, like gleams from the sun. Maybe they are trying to crack my mask and come back into my life. The mask is trapping me, but the orange is so close to me; just reach out and grab it. Pull it in.*

I put it away and went to lie back in bed. I wondered what my appointments would be like the next day. I had art therapy in the morning and then hypnotherapy in the afternoon. *What's hypnotherapy even about?* I knew I wouldn't like it, so what was the point of even going?

I wanted to watch a movie, an old movie that I hadn't seen in a while. I went to the VHS area of our movie cabinet and began searching through all the Disney movies. I made a pile of some that I was interested in watching and another pile that I didn't care about. When I got to the back of the shelf I noticed some bare VHS tapes, out of cases. One said "GA" on it. *Is it about me?* My mom and I sign things about me as "GA" because that's the state of Georgia's abbreviation.

I put it in the VHS player, but forgot what to do past that; *does this thing even work anymore?* I hadn't watched VHS for probably seven years, but I figured out how to get it started.

"Good morning, Georgia," I heard my dad whisper before I saw an image on the screen. "Hi, Georgia."

Then the black went away and I could see a little naked baby lying on my sleeping mom's chest. They were in the hospital. Then the phone rang. My mom woke up and the baby's eyes opened a little. She reached over and picked up the phone, "Hello?... Oh, hi!... Yeah, everything's fine; she's perfect... Georgia, Georgia Roxanne Huston... Doesn't it?..." The TV went black again.

It came back on after a few seconds, showing what I assumed was my parents' previous home; it had all the same paintings and furniture, but different rooms. I could see my mom holding the camera in the reflection of a mirror. I had no idea what my mom was wearing, it was a crazy outfit, but she looked so young and happy. Her hair was longer and thicker and her eyes were brighter.

My dad came into the room holding the baby; his hair wasn't gray.

He brought the baby over to the couch where I recognized my grandpa and handed her to him. My grandpa smiled and looked down at this baby, his first grandchild, and even though they had just met, he loved that baby with all his heart.

Then another woman came into the room, and I had absolutely no idea who she was. I racked my brain, but she didn't look familiar.

"Let me see," she ordered, walking quickly and effortlessly to the couch. She took the baby out of my grandpa's arms and looked down at it herself. She got lost in the innocence of the baby's face and for a moment it seemed like she had forgotten where she was.

"Ma, let me see you with her," my mom said, bringing the camera closer, snapping the woman holding the baby out of her trance. The woman looked up and smiled at the camera; it was my grandma.

She had dark hair and she was as plump as she could be, which is one reason I didn't recognize her. Another is that I had never really seen her like that. I didn't think that I had ever seen her moving around without the aid of a walker or wheelchair, and if I had, then it was many years ago. I had never thought of her as mobile, and seeing this woman on the screen, it hadn't even occur to me that it was her.

Everyone looked so young and happy on the screen. They all had a glow about them that I had never really seen. I turned off the TV before I had to watch anymore. I wiped my eyes, but more tears just came out. Everyone was smiling and walking around like something incredible had just happened; like they had just been blessed with a gift.

What they didn't know was that the innocent little baby they were admiring wasn't a gift at all. It was a curse and it was in their best interests to send it down the Nile River because nothing but heartache would come from that baby's life. It would become the biggest burden they would ever have to experience.

I am the burden. I am the baby that everyone had such hope and high expectations for. I am the baby that didn't deserve the unconditional love and support I received from my family and friends because I ended up just throwing it back into their faces. Their plan backfired and instead of having that beautiful baby girl grow up and be someone special, she turned into a liability.

I was crying my eyes out, wondering where I had gone; how I, their pride and joy, could turn around and be so awful to them.

How could I ruin their lives like this?

Chapter Twenty-three

I woke up in the laundry room, next to a huge pile of soft clothes, on the hard tile floor. I opened my eyes and my dad was standing over me, looking very concerned. "What happened?"

"I don't know, dad," I whispered, cringing as a shooting pain ran down my back. My arms and legs were numb, and after the pain subsided, my back was numb, too. *Oh shit.*

"What's wrong?" he asked in response to my grimacing face.

I took a deep breath so I wouldn't freak out when I said, "I can't move."

"Is it like before?"

"Kind of."

"Do you think you're okay?"

"I don't know, just let me be," I whispered with my eyes closed; *I can't be calm when you're drilling me with questions.*

"Dr. Nineteen gave me a muscle relaxer to give to you; do you want me to get it?" he said getting up.

"No, no dad. Just let me be."

I could hear him take a step back, but I still didn't want to open my eyes. *If I can't see the world, they can't see me. That means I'm not on the floor in my laundry room, I'm floating in the ocean. There is a nice breeze and the warm sun is beating down on me as I drift away on the calm, open waters. It doesn't matter where it takes me, as long as it's far away from the laundry room in the back corner of my house.*

After a half hour of not being able to move, feeling started to come back into my hands and arms. Again, my feet and legs were the last things to feel normal, but I waited patiently; I knew the drill. When I was comfortable enough to get up, my dad helped me back to bed.

To find our way back, all we had to do was to follow my path of destruction. Some things were knocked off the dining room table and there was a chair on its side in the living room. My knees were all banged up from running into things. But no matter how many things I ran into or knocked over, the thing that I was really bruising was my self-esteem.

Slow down, you're doing fine
You can't be everything you want to be
Before your time
Although it's so romantic on the borderline tonight...

I can't help what speed I'm going, I'm usually not even conscious when I'm moving around. Doing fine, Billy? Do you really call this doing fine? Look at my knees, my elbows, and my forehead; bruises. The bruises are from running into that table, and that wall over there – I am not doing fine, don't lie to me. I always knew that I couldn't be "everything" I wanted to be, but now I know that I can't be anything I want to be. I am a nobody and that's all I am ever going to be; before my time, during my time, or after my time – it doesn't make a difference. Romantic is not exactly the word that I would use to describe tonight. I'd go with nightmare. I would agree that I am on the borderline tonight – the borderline of my sanity, or what's left of it anyway. Every time I look in the mirror it gets harder and harder to recognize myself.

"Where are the places today?" I asked my dad in the car on the way to my first art therapy appointment.
"They are both over the hill like Beth's," he answered. *Great, more long car rides.*
"Did you really have to bring my art portfolio?" I asked eyeing the pile of art in the back seat.
"Georgia, she's an artist who is going to be doing art with you. Doesn't it make sense to show her some of your work?"

Esther's office was in a very happening part of town. It was really hard to find parking and there was crazy traffic on her street; welcome to Beverly Hills. Her building was on the older side and the elevator really intimidated me. I have a hard time riding in elevators anyway, but that creaky one always made me nervous. *Hopefully I'll be well enough to take the stairs soon.*
Her door was the first one you see when the elevator doors open. *Do we just walk in?* My dad started to open the door. "Wait," I said, "knock first." He rolled his eyes and opened the door for me .
I walked into a really small waiting room with two leather chairs. It

was dimly lit, had nice soft music playing in the background, and had a lot of books. It was very stylish and artsy, but that wasn't unexpected.

As soon as we sat down in the leather armchairs, the door opened and a woman with dark straight hair popped her head in. "Georgia?" she asked, with the heaviest German accent that I have ever heard in person.

"Yes," I smiled.

"Come on in," she said holding the door open.

"Do I come in, too?" my dad asked.

"Yes."

The inside of her office was awesome. One wall was windows, looking out over the busy street, one wall was all red brick, and the other two were a calm teal color. All of her furniture was very sleek. My dad and I sat on the couch and she sat facing us in another leather armchair.

"I'm Esther. Are you Georgia's father?"

"Yes, I am. I'm Jimmy."

"Tell me a little about yourself," she said to me.

"Well," I said pointing to my dad, "he says it best."

When will it end? Will I ever be at a part in my life where I could introduce myself and not have to explain my life story? Where they could just meet me and not my horrible past? Can they know me for me and not for all my awful experiences?

"…but we brought some of her art with us today," he finished, handing her the stack of artwork.

"Oh," she said looking through it, "this is very nice."

"Thanks," I smiled.

"Unfortunately," she continued looking through my portfolio, "we don't have any time today to do art — but we will next time for sure. Is that okay?"

Had it really been an hour of my dad talking?

"That's fine."

We had two hours to kill before my hypnotherapy appointment, so my dad and I went to Mulberry Pizza across the street from Esther's. It was a really small place, but every single one of its white walls was absolutely covered with pictures, messages, and signatures. It was fun to look around at all the famous people who had been in this tiny pizzeria.

I wanted to make my mark, but I knew nothing would come of it. No one knew who I was and no one wanted to. I couldn't make a mark on the wall, in the world, or even in my own life. I had no importance anywhere.

When we drove down the hypnotherapist's street I could tell right away which house was hers. There was a Japanese garden theme in her front yard that was very relaxing, that really stuck out in that neighborhood. *What did I get myself into?*

We walked along the stepping stones and pushed the doorbell. A very nice blonde lady opened the door. "Hi! Come on in," she smiled.

"Thanks," my dad said as we followed her inside.

"You must be Georgia," she said shaking my hand.

"Yeah," I smiled politely back.

"And I'm Jimmy," my dad said, shaking her hand also.

"Nice to meet you both. Please come in," she said walking into her living room. "Have a seat."

It was a decent sized room, naturally lit by all the sun coming in through the blinds. There was a huge couch that ran around the wall of the room and a chair next to it. There was a piece of fabric covering what I expected to be a TV across from the couch. It was a nice friendly room that I could tell had a lot of fun memories with her family. It didn't look like an office, you could tell that this was her home.

When the three of us were settled in our seats she introduced herself. "My name is Kathryn and I have been working with UCLA for quite some time now. Do you know why we use hypnotherapy and how it helps kids with chronic pain?"

"Not at all," I said, relieved that I didn't have to ask.

"What our clinic tries to do is supply our kids – our kids meaning patients – with the tools that are essential to dealing with their pain. We have a lot of kids with a lot of different problems, and therefore have many different options that can be used as solutions. Just because Alice loves hypnotherapy but hates yoga doesn't mean that Fred will like hypnotherapy or dislike yoga. We realize that you are all individuals so there is no one prescription that we can write and say, 'Physical therapy and craniosacral massage is all you have to do to get better.' Everyone is different and it's up to you to decide what works best for you and what doesn't." She took a breath.

"The reason I'm telling you this is that the same way acupuncture or biofeedback isn't for everyone, neither is hypnotherapy. If you don't feel like this is helping you, please don't be afraid to tell me or Dr. Twenty-one. We are here to help you. Does that make sense?"

"Yes," I said.

"So what we are going to be doing here is trying to give you an escape from everything. We are going to be working on relaxation so that when you are in stressful situations or pain, you can come back to your tools and remember hypnotherapy. I have patients tell me how they almost had a panic attack when they were out with friends, but they used what I taught them to stop it and move on. That's our goal. Do you get panic attacks?" she asked.

"Yes, really bad ones," I answered.

"Speaking of that, let me tell you what has been going on with her," my dad interjected.

"Okay," she held up a finger and looked around for something. "Hold that thought. Let me get my notebook so I can take notes."

When she found it my dad started the tale; the tale of Georgia.

Once upon a time there was a beautiful princess named Georgia. She had amazing friends and lived a happy life full of excitement and adventure. One day the evil witch cast a horrible spell on her, cursing her with a new illness called "pain."

The princess was really scared, but so was everyone else. Her friends stopped being interested in her and her family got frustrated because while they tried to help, they couldn't. Princess Georgia was all alone and felt lost and confused. All she wanted was to be normal again... What happens next?

Will the evil witch get away with it, or will my fairy Godmother come to save me? I've got to have a fairy Godmother, don't I? Everyone has to have someone like that to protect them; where is mine?

"Well that just sounds awful," Kathryn said when my dad was done. "I hope I can help you." *Me, too.* "We don't have much time left, but if you want, we could do a little practice run. What do you think?"

Ugh. "I'd love to."

"Great, so Jimmy, if you wouldn't mind stepping out for a little bit?" she asked politely. He left. Now it was just Kathryn and me.

"So Georgia, you should get comfortable. If you want to sit in that black chair next to you, it reclines and might be more comfortable – it's your choice though."

I followed her advice, moved chairs, and reclined. "Okay, close your eyes and take deep breaths... deeper and deeper until you feel completely relaxed... feel yourself sinking deeper and deeper into your chair... listen to my voice..."

"So how'd it go?" my dad asked in the car on the way home.

"It was fine," I said. "We didn't have much time so we'll see how it goes next time. It was relaxing though."

So far I had no idea how all of these random things were going to tie together and help me out, if they were even going to.

Yeah, making art was fun, yoga felt good, and hypnotherapy relaxed me, but how are those supposed to stop my pain; my fake pain?

Maybe this is all an act. Maybe since this is my fake pain they are just telling me all of this to get in my head. They are trying to trick me! Since it's fake, if I believe that this stuff, these stupid "therapies," are going to help, won't they? That's smart of them. They have figured out a system of making us do useless things in order to push the pain out of our minds. If we believe we are getting better, we will – because it's all fake.

"How'd it go today?" my mom asked, lying down in the bed next to me.

"It was fine," I answered staring at the TV. My back was hurting so badly that I was fighting back tears.

"Yeah?" she asked excitedly, trying to engage me. "Tell me about it."

"I really don't want to right now." *Just go away; leave me alone.*

"Did you do any art in art therapy?" she politely persisted.

"No, mom," I whined, hinting that I didn't want to talk.

"What was hypnotherapy like?" she asked, losing some of her enthusiasm but still trying.

The pain throbbed and I strained every muscle in my body out of reflex. I felt my legs starting to cramp due to how tense my muscles were.

I winced but she didn't see. "I don't know, mom!" I snapped.

"Okay," she said after a pause. She pretended she wasn't hurt, but I could tell that she really was. "I'm gonna go say 'hi' to your sister and then make dinner." She got up sulking and left the room.

No mom! Come back, I'm so sorry. I love you so much. Today was actually really interesting and it was great meeting all the people that Dr. Twenty-one raved about at our appointment. They all seem like really genuine people and I look forward to spending more time with them. We didn't have time to do anything in art therapy today since it was kind of a meet-and-greet. She said we would do some next time. Hypnotherapy was also just getting to know each other, but she seems to have a lot of hope that she can help me. We did a little exercise today but, just like with Esther, we are going to be doing more next time. And about before, I'm so sorry. I'm really having a hard time right now, but I shouldn't have taken it out on you. I'm sorry and I love that you are so interested in my day. You are the best mom ever and I love you so much.

I wanted to say so much to her, I wanted her to come back so I could make it right.

Why do I keep messing up? If I keep this up, even fewer people are going to want to help me.

I hurt anything and anyone who comes in my path. I am like an earthquake; you think everything's fine and then when you least expect it, I shake your world in every direction possible. I throw your beloved picture frames and china on the floor and crush them into millions of pieces. I break the pipes under your house so water comes in and floods your floors. I break the gate for your front yard and your dog runs away. I am the earthquake that everyone dreads and thinks they are prepared for, but when I come into your life I always make a bigger impact than you expect. I am destruction, I am devastation; I am pain.

I need to stop turning people away who just want the best for me; they just want to help.

Chapter Twenty-four

I woke up to my mom and dad holding me down. Every muscle in my body ached and I was exhausted. When they saw my eyes open they both relaxed and took deep breaths. It was pitch dark outside and the movie I had on the TV was over. *How long was I out?*

Words cannot express how scary it is to have blackouts and not have any recollection of what happened. Blackouts are one thing, waking up to your parents' disturbed expressions is another. Waking up and knowing that your body did something that you are not aware of – that is completely horrifying. Imagine knowing that you just did something, something to get everyone else's attention, but you don't know what; that's the real nightmare.

Since I was doing strange things in my sleep, including bolting out of bed while everyone else was asleep, my parents decided they were going to both sleep with me from now on. *Finally Veronica will get the big bed she's always wanted.*

My mom slept on my left and my dad slept on my right. When my dad was asleep he would always keep one arm over me so when I got up unconsciously or seized, the movement would wake him up. It was annoying to have his arm on me all night, especially since I barely got any sleep, but I knew it was necessary. I was hurting myself in my sleep. I was crazy; I was dangerous.

I woke up to a new, beautiful day… with nothing to do. *It's second period at school right now; I would've been in my art class.*

"Good morning, Peaches." My mom came in like nothing had happened the night before; like nothing was wrong.

"Hi mom," I said awkwardly.

"So tonight Dawn and everyone are coming over for dinner. I just wanted to give you a heads up."

"Is Talia coming?"

"As far as I know," she shrugged. It was always a treat when Talia came. She was older than us, so she had more things to do. It was always a pleasant surprise when she came, too.

"Are we going to go out?"

"Yeah, I don't know where yet, though."

A couple of hours went by of being by myself, and then a few more. I took out my phone and started looking through my contacts. I couldn't find anyone I wanted to text because I already knew no one wanted to talk to me; no one wanted to be bothered by me. I was a burden.

I spent the day staring at the ceiling, petting my dogs, and then staring at the ceiling some more; that's all that my days really consisted of. There was no substance in my life anymore. All I had was solitude.

Humans are not supposed to be alone, I learned over time. We are naturally social beings and we are like that for a reason. Through being social we learn more and experience more, which is why being able to communicate with people is so important in this world. Human interaction is crucial to our success and happiness, and that's just the way it is.

In prisons, isolation is used as a form of punishment. If prisoners misbehave, they might be sent to solitary confinement. They are stuck in there without any human interaction at all. They can't even see the people who bring their meals. It is an awful experience that can torment one's mind. Interrogators often use solitary confinement as a method to break down their subjects because it is such a severe experience.

Historically, society's serial killers and sociopaths were usually also society's outcasts. If they didn't develop mental problems due to their isolation, it did build up resentment, which could lead to their horrific actions. People need to feel accepted and need to belong to some sort of class. Maybe that is a flaw in our society, putting pressures on people that shouldn't be there, or maybe it's just the nature of mankind.

Am I being tortured? Did I do some awful thing that I don't remember or maybe didn't even realize I did? If I did, I'm sorry; I'm so so sorry. Maybe this is karma, maybe I deserve this, but for whatever reason this is happening to me, please know that I will do anything to be forgiven.

What's going to happen to me? Am I going to turn into a sociopath? Am I going to just crack one of these days and have some atrocious reaction to what my life has become? What if I hurt people? Am I capable of that? Who wouldn't be after all this? What if I do something awful while I am unconscious? Can I be held accountable for that? What if I go to jail for something I didn't even mean to do? My defense: I have a made up pain in my head that's driving me crazy.

It was pure torture for me to be isolated. I got to experience first-hand all the tricks that someone's mind plays on them when they are alone for long periods of time. When it is just you alone, you have no true sense of reality because we use other people's reactions to show us what's real and what's not, what's true versus false. The reason I knew that green was green was because everyone told me that. If I didn't have someone to tell me, I would have a completely different perception of what the color green was. People need other people for guidance and verification; I didn't have that.

"Jaja!" Sarah jumped on me and woke me up.

"Hey Sare," I opened my eyes and smiled.

"Hi Georgia," Talia came in. Dawn and Steve followed.

"Oh hey," I smiled, sitting up.

"Oh no," Dawn shooed me to lie back down. "Don't get up."

"No it's fine, I want to. I've been lying down all day," I said slowly standing up. "Can you please hand me my crutches?"

"How are you doing?" Apateece asked in a goofy voice, giving me a hug.

"Not great," I answered.

Dawn gave me a hug next, "We brought a cherry pie."

I laughed, "You guys know us so well."

My family came out when they heard them.

"So where do you guys want to go?" my dad asked.

"I'll have anything," Talia said.

"Me, too," Dawn agreed.

"Steve?" my dad asked.

He shrugged, "Whatever you want," but I knew he probably wanted Mexican food.

"What do you want, Georgia?" Dawn asked me politely.

"Pizza?" I said.

"Pizza it is," she said, enthusiastically standing up.

I knew my dad wasn't happy with that decision, but he went along with it. "Can you walk?" he asked.

The pizza place we always went to was only two blocks away. I had walked there a million and ten times; *of course I can walk there.* "Yeah," I said crutching to the door. "Let's go."

We passed the awkward house with only two windows, and the house with the fence that doesn't match the rest of the house. We passed the place where I fell off my scooter with Jordan and scraped my knee, and the new house that was just built. It was my first time walking around the neighborhood in a while and it felt different. It felt like a *deja vu* of a dream, but I knew it wasn't; it was memory of a past life.

I was struggling a little on the walk, but I hid it well. I worked so hard to keep up and not show how difficult it was for me, because while it was hard, it wasn't unmanageable. I was relieved when I saw the shining lights of "Robbie Mac's Pizza," and smelled the amazing food that was waiting for me inside.

I always ordered two slices of olive pizza. I'd eat one there and bring the second one home to eat the next day, and either a lemonade or a Sierra Mist. When we'd all ordered and were settled at our table, I knew it was time for the drilling.

"How have you been feeling lately?... What did the doctor say?... Has it been getting worse?..."

I knew they were just showing concern, which I appreciated, but at the same time I didn't want it. I wanted to be normal.

As soon as everyone finished with their pizza, I had an idea. "Can we go to Handmade?" I asked. Handmade was a store a few doors down that was really cool and fun to visit.

"In a couple of minutes," my dad said.

"No, I mean just us," I hinted.

He thought about it. "Can't you just wait for us?"

"Dad, please." This wasn't just about going to the store. It was about having semi-independence, even if it was just for five minutes.

He finally agreed. "If Talia and Veronica feel comfortable with it."

While we were walking to Handmade I started to realize how risky this was. I got nervous, thinking about all the awful things that could happen and my dad wasn't going to be there to protect me. *Have I become like a little kid again?* I felt so lost and vulnerable in my own neighborhood, just because I wasn't with my dad; *how sad.*

We ended up having a lot of fun shopping and looking around. Talia got a pair of red vintage boots and I got some candy. It was fun to feel like a regular teenager for a little bit, but it was also scary; I was out of my comfort zone. *I am out in a situation that I would have done with such ease a year ago. This pain has impacted and changed my life so drastically that it might have also altered my personality. What if I'm not the same person anymore?*

Walking back home with everyone was extremely difficult. On top of my pain being awful, I was a lot more tired than before. I would go really slowly, struggling to stay upright, and then I would have bursts of speed where I would be ahead of everyone because I wanted to get it over with. I was secretly crying as the pads cut into my armpits and my shoulders cramped. I was falling apart in front of everyone. *Maybe I shouldn't go out of the house anymore.*

When we finally got back home I was out of breath and exhausted. As soon as my dad unlocked the front door I flew through it and collapsed on the mattresses on the floor and closed my eyes.

"Georgia!" My mom screamed and lunged for me.

"Mom, I'm fine," I said rudely.

"Did you pass out?"

"No." *When did it become a crime to just close my eyes? I can close them of my own free will, too. It doesn't just happen when I pass out.*

Then, as they all filed through the door and spread out around the living room, I did pass out.

I woke up to laughter, dancing, and the piano playing. Sarah and Veronica were dancing, with Sarah copying all Veronica's moves. Talia and my mom were pounding away at the piano like they usually did. Dawn and Steve were laughing at them and telling them how to dance.

"Are you okay?" My dad was lying right next to me, staring at me with concern.

"Yeah," I said faking a yawn, "I just fell asleep." He knew I was lying, but he let it go.

"Jaja, dance!" Sarah shrieked happily and ran up to me. She took my arm and tried to pull me up, but I shook my head.

"I can just dance here, Sare," I said moving my arms and head around like I was dancing.

"No," she laughed and continued to pull at me. "Come dance with me and Nakka!"

"I'm sorry, baby," I said letting go of her hand. "I can't."

"Sare Sare," Talia said walking over to her. "Leave Georgia alone, come on baby." Talia sat on the bed. "What do you want to do?"

"Not much I can do," I said.

"Let's play cards." She got up without seeing if I wanted to and went into my room. She returned with my cards and plopped back down on the mattress.

"Oh, I want to play," Veronica said and sat down with us.

"Me, too!" Sarah followed.

"Okay Sarah, you can be on my team," I said and she sat on my lap. I winced. I was having a hard time sitting up because my pain was so bad, but I fought through it.

"What are we going to play?" Talia asked shuffling the cards.

"Gin," Veronica answered.

"Georgia," Talia looked at me, "what do you want to play?"

I shrugged, "Gin's fine." Gin was my grandpa's game and we always played it with him. It was a big day when one of us would occasionally beat him because he was a master. But, if you play someone who's a master, you also get pretty good. Veronica and I were pretty good at Gin. I knew with grandpa's help, Sarah was going to be, too, one day.

"Who goes first?" Veronica asked.

"Me!" Sarah raised her hand.

"Okay," Talia laughed. "Sarah and Jaja go first."

"I can't do it today," I said crying to my dad.

"Georgia," he said trying to calm me. "Is it the pain or are you just down?"

"Everything! My life sucks and I hate it so much." I felt like a toddler having a tantrum, but I really didn't care; I needed to let steam out.

"Your life doesn't suck," he lied through his teeth.

"Stop, don't you dare tell me that. Don't you start lying to me, too!"

"You know you are going to get through this."

"How the hell can you even tell me that right now?!" I raised my voice.

"Because it's true," he said desperately.

"No, no it's not. No one knows what's wrong with me and no one knows what to do." I flung my head back, which hurt my back so I screamed and threw a pillow over my face, crying my eyes out.

"We don't 'not know' anymore, Georgia. We do know what's going on. This doctor knows what's going on and she's going to help you."

"No dad, she is not going to help. Are you really that blind? Do you really not know what's going to happen here? She is just going to become another chapter in my book, another doctor who threw up her hands at me. She is just going to be another person who gave up on me."

"You can't think like that if you want to get better," he interrupted.

"It's not about getting better anymore. I don't even know what it's about. There's no reason to get better because there is no way I can get better. There is no hope for me anymore."

No hope? Is that really how I feel?

Chapter Twenty-five

I peered secretly through the blinds, watching my dad walk him in. He was carrying something really big with him. I laid back down and pretended I had been there the whole time.

"Georgia, this is Chris," my dad said.

"Hi Georgia," Chris smiled and shook my hand.

"Hi," I smiled back.

"I'll let you guys get to work," my dad said and left the room.

"So Georgia, do you understand what I do?" Chris asked, unfolding the big thing that he was carrying; a massage table.

"You massage me?" *It's pretty self-explanatory.*

He smiled, "It's a special kind of massage. It's called craniosacral massage and it's not the kind of massage that most people get. I'm not going to be rubbing or anything like that. I'm going to be pressing, to find your pressure points and areas of stress and push them out using positive energy and light touches or stretches. It doesn't hurt at all."

Doesn't sound like much of a massage. "Will I be sore after?"

"I don't think so," he answered, taking out a couple of sheets and folding them on the massage table. Then he took out his Ipod and plugged it into some portable speakers he'd brought. "Where's the light switch?"

I pointed to the wall and he dimmed the lights.

"If you want, you can lie down on the table." Then he got his Ipod and turned on relaxing music.

I had never had a professional massage before, so I just went by what I saw in the movies. I lay face down so he could have easy access to my back. "I'm actually going to have you lie on your back," he said.

How is that going to work?

I obliged and sank deep into the massage table. But, it wasn't a table exactly; it was a Tempur-Pedic massage table, which made it extremely comfortable. He put a pillow under my head. It felt like a beanbag chair with all the little beads in it conforming to my head.

"I have some oils that smell good. Would you like one?" he offered.

"Sure," I shrugged.

"Which one do you want?" he asked, showing me the box.

I read through them. "Can I have lavender?"

He smiled, "Of course." He took the little bottle out and poured some on his finger. "I'm going to put it on your neck, okay?"

"That's fine."

As soon as he dabbed it on my neck I smelled the strong scent of lavender. I coughed at first, but after a few seconds I got used to it and actually enjoyed it. It relaxed me.

He brought one of the dining room chairs over to my left side. He put a sheet over me, so I was between two sheets. "Close your eyes," he said softly, "listen to the music and smell the lavender."

I did what he told me to do. I took deep breaths and tried to relax my body. He slipped his hands under my back, but still had a sheet in between his hand and my back. *I don't have cooties!* He went around my back, just touching it ever so softly. *Was this the massage?* He would occasionally press harder in some areas, but even his "harder" was super-gentle. When he was done with the left side of my back, he went to my right side. After that he went down my legs, pushing on different areas, and he pulled my feet to stretch out my legs. Then he rolled and stretched my neck and massaged my head while the scent of lavender massaged my nostrils.

I was in an unfamiliar state of mind. I could feel Chris's gentle hands moving around my body and I could smell the lavender, but I couldn't hear the music or move. It was like part of my consciousness was there and the other part wasn't. I was somewhere in the middle of being awake and being asleep. I wasn't even able to think. It was like both my mind and body were paralyzed. It was an incredibly comforting feeling to be lost in my own mind.

When he was done, my heart sank as I floated back to reality. The reality was that it wasn't just my mind and the lavender; it was me in my living room in front of my mattress on the floor. In front of me was the TV where I watched countless useless shows, and to my left was the window that I would stare out and watch life continue on while I was stuck inside. Even the plants in my yard had a better life than me. At least they got to enjoy the sunshine and feel the breeze. They were healthy and they got to grow.

I wanted to be healthy. I wanted to know what it's like to hang out with my friends and not have to worry about holding them back because of my physical restrictions. I wanted to sleep during normal sleeping hours and stay awake while everyone else was. I wanted to not be doped up on drugs and keep reality separate from the craziness of my chaotic thoughts and delusions. I wanted to just see one doctor a year for my yearly checkup; no more doctors but that one a year.

I wanted to grow. I wanted to be as tall as the trees and as fruitful as the bushes. I wanted everyone to notice me when I came into a room and they had to move out of my way or else they would get stepped on. I wanted to be in control of everything. I wanted to be so tall that I soaked up all the sun so I could grow even more. I wanted to grow in knowledge, too. If someone looked at me I wanted them to see how smart I was, just like the rings on a tree show how old it is. I wanted my wisdom to be known and to be respected. All I wanted was to be healthy and grow like the trees in my yard. *How sad is that? I envy a tree.*

Stop snoring in my ear! My dad was on my right with his arm around me and my mom was on my left. Nights were awful for me because I was always in so much pain and so tense that I could never relax enough to really fall asleep. Everyone around me would be asleep and I would just lie there and wait for the sun to come in through the blinds.

I was flipping through the TV channels and saw that "Ferris Bueller's Day Off" was on. I recorded it to watch later, but after finding that there was nothing else I wanted to see, I turned that on. I'd only seen that movie once and it was years before. I didn't remember much about it.

It's about a high school kid who pretends that he's sick so he can stay home from school, and then has an amazing adventure with his friends. I wanted to be like Ferris. *Who wouldn't want to be like him?*

It's not so much the adventure that I wanted, I wanted to be able to pretend like I was sick and then take off my mask and be perfectly fine. I wanted to be carefree and spontaneous, like Ferris. I wanted to be well.

Ferris Bueller became my only real comfort at night. When everyone fell asleep I would watch that movie over and over again. I would never get sick of that movie. I tried to live through his day as much as possible and do all those outrageous things with him; *only in the movies.*

I woke up with my sweaty dad holding me down with all his might; his face was bright red. When I opened my eyes and saw how much he was struggling I just started crying. *How much longer can he do this? He was holding me down like he was holding on for his own life.*

But he is holding on for his own life. I have become his life in a larger sense than children should be for their parents. He has gone into protection mode and he won't stop trying until it kills him. I am going to be the death of my poor dad.

"I'll be right back," he said. He came back a couple of minutes later and said, "Barbara's coming over."

"Who's Barbara?" I asked. The only Barbara I could think of was my aunt Barbara who lived in Athens, Georgia.

"Kelsey's mom."

Kelsey was one of Veronica's teammates and friends; *why would her mom be coming over?* "Why?"

"She's gonna spend some time with you." *Umm... okay? You're making me playdates with grown women?*

Barbara came right over and was very nice. She sat on the mattress with me, down on the living room floor.

"What do you want to do?" she asked. *Oh my God, she really is my playdate.*

"I don't know. What do you want to do?" *How awkward.*

"Whatever you want." She thought for a second. "Do you like games?"

"I like Monopoly," I smiled.

"Monopoly it is." She slapped the bed playfully. "Where is it?"

"Right there." I pointed to the box next to the couch; out and ready, as usual. "I call being the shoe."

Getting lost in the game of Monopoly was one of my favorite things to do. I ruled the board and everyone knew it. People would come in cocky, and then I'd blow their socks off; it was great. In the game of Monopoly I had control.

When we finished the game (I of course won), I had a seizure. I woke up to Barbara on top of me that time, exhausted and out of breath. She was a strong lady so she held me down pretty well.

"Can you get my dad?" I asked awkwardly.

"What do you need?" she answered sitting up.

"I'm thirsty," I lied.

"What do you want, I'll get it." She stood up.

"No, Barbara, it's fine. My dad can get it," I insisted.

"Let's give your dad a break," she said nicely. "What do you want?"

That's why she was there, to give my dad a break. My dad called her because he needed a break from being my dad. He needed a break from me.

Chapter Twenty-Six

"So how's Notre Dame going?" my grandpa asked.
"I haven't been going, remember?" I said.
"Still?" he seemed surprised. "Is it because of those crutches?"
"Yeah," I lied. *How would he understand what chronic pain was if I didn't even understand it? I didn't want him to know the truth; that his first grandchild was crazy.*
"So you haven't been able to play softball?"
"No," I reminded him, "it's not softball season."
"Oh, that's right," he remembered. "I'm gonna come to one of your games though."
"I know you are grandpa."
"When you're on the Notre Dame team – when you're winning all the games for them."
"Okay, I'll keep an eye out for you."

That day when I got home, my dad handed me a big envelope from Notre Dame. I opened it anxiously to find a stack of about forty cards, all addressed to me. Everyone in my algebra class had written me a 'get well' card. It made me so happy that they remembered me and that they were thinking of me. I felt very supported.

I shivered. Esther's office was always cold.
"So how has your week been?" We were sitting across from each other; I was on the couch and she was in the armchair.
"It's been good," I was not in the mood to have a shrink.
"What'd you do?"
"Nothing really." *Can we just do some art now?*
"You didn't go out at all?"
I thought about it. "I saw my grandparents, but that was about it."
"Oh, and how are they doing?"

"Good." I was being difficult on purpose because I just wanted to get to the fun stuff.

"Do you want to come over to the desk so we can start a project?" She nodded at the desk against the wall.

Yes! "Sure," I shrugged.

When she got all the utensils and we both got settled in, she looked at me and said, "For this project I want you to draw a self-portrait."

"Just a self-portrait?"

She smiled. "Just a self-portrait."

"Can I have a mirror?"

"No," she laughed. "I don't want that kind of self-portrait. I want you to draw what you think you look like."

Of course I knew what I looked like, but when I had to really focus and try to remember everything, it proved to be a bigger challenge than I had thought. I knew my drawing was not going to be very accurate at all; *great, the first art I show her is going to be horrible. She's going to think I'm a terrible artist.* I knew I just had to go for it; *draw what you think you look like.*

I looked at the box of pastels in front of me and took out the blue one. I drew the outline of a face and nose with the blue pastel, but didn't color the face in. I used the black and red pastels to draw my eyes and gray to outline my mouth. I colored my mouth in with orange and then drew my hair and eyebrows a normal brown. *Great,* it doesn't look anything like me.

"I know it's not good." I was disappointed. "Can I start over?"

"No, no," she said. "It's great. I like it a lot." She held it up and looked at it closer. "Can you tell me about it?"

"What do you mean?"

"Why did you make your self-portrait this way?" She leaned the picture against the wall so I could see it.

"Do you mean like the colors or what?"

"Sure, tell me about the colors."

I thought about it. "The blue outlining means that I am sad and depressed. The red and black eyes show how frustrated and angry I am. The mouth is outlined in gray, but colored orange because I have a lot to say, but I can't say it."

"Why can't you say it?"

"I don't know."

"Is it that you can't say it, or that you won't say it?"

"Won't say it."

On the way home I really started to think about my self-portrait and how that wasn't someone that I wanted to be. I don't want to have anger and frustration in my eyes, or sadness outlining my face; I didn't want to be afraid to say anything. *I want my old self back.*

I remembered what Dr. Twenty-one had said before. She told me to get on with my life and that was exactly what I was going to do. I was going to go on living because I had so much more to offer the world. I was meant for more than an orange mouth with a gray outline.

"Georgia?" My dad came in the living room with my mom following him. "Can you turn off the TV for a second?"

I turned it off. I started to get butterflies in my stomach. They both sat down on either side of me.

"We have something to tell you," he started.

"But everything's going to be okay," my mom interrupted. Every moment that went by I got more and more freaked out. *What else could go wrong in my life?*

"Yes," my dad agreed, "everything's going to be okay." I wanted to ask what was going on, but I was too scared to find out. "Notre Dame contacted us… They want you to withdraw from school."

My eyes started to tear up. "What do you mean?"

"I mean they want us to formally take you out of school," he said solemnly, "but they said they will hold your spot for next year."

"How am I going to go there next year if I don't finish my ninth grade?" I asked, fighting back my hyperventilating.

"We will figure it out," my mom said hugging me.

"Can you guys leave me alone for a little?" I said as calmly as I could.

"But honey..." my mom started, but my dad signaled for her to leave.

When I was alone I put on Billy, threw the blankets over my head, and started sobbing.

Too bad but it's the life you lead
you're so ahead of yourself that you forgot what you need
Though you can see when you're wrong, you know
You can't always see when you're right. You're right…

I don't lead a life; everyone else leads it for me. How can I be ahead of anyone, including myself, at this point? I can't do anything. I haven't forgotten what I need; I know exactly what I need; that's not the problem. The problem is actually getting what I need. I'm always wrong, never right, and that's all there is to it. I'm always doing something wrong.

Not Notre Dame; anything but Notre Dame. I can't let someone else down and have yet another person tell me that they don't want to be involved with me. Even though I wasn't going to school or being a part of it, I still felt like I had a home there. I felt like I was welcomed there, but I'm not; yet another person to turn their back on me.

I wonder what they are going to say about me at school, other than the things they are already saying. The rumors about me are probably awful. I will never be able to show my face there again. Well, not to worry, they are making sure that I won't have to. Maybe this is a good thing; maybe they are taking the pain and humiliation out of this for me. No, who am I kidding? This is the worst thing that could have happened to me. Am I going to have to retake ninth grade as a tenth grader? Will I ever go back to Notre Dame? What's going to happen to me?

I had to fight back a panic attack; *I can't go through another one.* I took deep breaths and closed my eyes; I could feel my hot breath being pushed back into my face by the blanket two inches away from my mouth. I was sweating bullets and my breathing started to get faster and faster. I put Billy on louder, but I couldn't even hear him serenading me over my loud heartbeat.

Notre Dame doesn't want me anymore; no one does. I knew I had to calm down, but for some reason I couldn't.

Should I call for my dad? No, there's nothing he can do. All it would do was worry him.

I felt like I was on my own for now. I wanted to see if I could calm myself down without anyone's help, not that anyone could really help.

I started to see spots and I was getting really dizzy. I was hyperventilating too much, *but how am I supposed to stop it?* There was nothing I could do as I just lay there helplessly, losing crucial oxygen. *I'm going to die here.* My legs and arms were cramping and I was in excruciating pain before I lost consciousness.

I didn't know if I passed out because of too much carbon dioxide under the blanket with me, or if I just did my usual passing out. I didn't know if I'd had a seizure while I was unconscious or if I just lay still. I was a little disoriented when I woke up, but soon felt reality flood back into my mind. I was back; back to my sucky life.

A couple of days went by of utter depression. I didn't want to get up for anything; *there's no reason to anyway.* I didn't know when it was night or when it was day, the blinds were always shut and the lights were always off. I stayed awake, but I wasn't truly awake. I was in a zombie-like state that was hard to explain to my family. It was like I was spacing out the whole time and while I could see and hear things, I couldn't really process them. *I have never been so down in my life,* but then I remembered that I had thought that many times before.

How much worse is my life going to get? It seemed like every time I started to feel hopeful, something new came along. It felt like I wasn't just getting the rug pulled out from under me, but I was also getting stepped on and kicked, only to have the rug put back over me. The rug was being stapled down on the floor with me still under it and there was nothing I could do.

"I can't do that," I told my upside down yoga instructor. She was hanging from a rope on the wall, with all her body weight, and didn't look nervous at all.

"Yes you can," she laughed getting down and out of the rope. "We'll walk through it." She wrapped a blanket around my waist. "Put your legs on the wall, right here," she said, putting the rope around my butt. "Now lean back."

"No." I looked at her like she was crazy.

"Why not?"

"Do you see how thin these ropes are and how big I am? How the heck are these little ropes screwed into the wall going to hold me?"

"Georgia," Beth laughed, "they are not going to break. Do you know how many people, of all shapes and sizes, have hung from these ropes? Too many to count, and I have never had any rope break. Trust me and just lean back."

I weighed the pros and cons in my mind. "Do you promise?"

"I promise."

Leaning on those ropes felt like skydiving out of an airplane for me. It was nerve racking, but I didn't fall. I put my legs up the wall and let my head dangle freely and after a while I got pretty comfortable; it was actually kind of fun.

"So how have you been doing?" Beth asked sitting down on the floor next to me.

"Not good," I answered.

"Why not?" She seemed genuinely concerned. "You can tell me anything."

"I've just been feeling really depressed and stressed lately, especially since I got kicked out of school."

"What have you been doing to deal with the stress?"

"Having panic attacks and passing out," I said sarcastically.

"But really Georgia, you have to learn how to deal with it. Have you tried yoga when you're having a panic attack?"

I laughed, but then stopped when I saw that she was serious. "I don't have ropes like this at home," I said to save myself.

"You don't need ropes. What about all the other poses we've been doing?"

"I can barely move during panic attacks, much less strike a yoga pose."

"Are you relaxed when you're doing them?"

"Yeah."

"Then try it next time. There's no harm in trying."

"Okay, I'll try."

After a pause she asked me, "Do you know what a mantra is?"

"No, what is it?"

"It's like a prayer. For example, one Hindu mantra is, 'May prosperity be glorified, may rulers rule the world with law and justice, may divinity and erudition be protected. May all beings be happy and prosperous.' It's like a prayer and it calms you down, giving you a moment to reflect on what you are feeling. Maybe you could find a mantra online somewhere and use it when you're stressed," she suggested.

"Yeah, that's a good idea. I'll look into that."

"It's time to come out now," she said, "so carefully walk your legs down the wall and slowly come out… that's right, now lean your head against the wall so the blood can circulate a little before you stand up."

My eyes were closed and my forehead was on the wall as I waited for my head to feel normal again. "Beth?" I asked. "Does this stuff really work?"

"What stuff?" she asked, folding my blanket.

"Dr. Twenty-one's tools for chronic pain or whatever?"

She put her hand on my shoulder. "I wouldn't be here if it didn't."

"Can you sign this?" My dad handed me a piece of paper.

"What is it?" I asked, taking the pen from his hand.

He took a deep breath. "The withdrawal forms for Notre Dame. I'm taking them back to the office this afternoon."

Without reading it I just signed it, tears in my eyes. I didn't want to read it; I knew what it said. I wanted to just sign it so he could get it out of my face; I wanted to forget about it. With each stroke of the pen I could feel myself falling deeper and deeper into a hole. I was losing myself; I was signing my soul away, but I didn't have a choice.

I knew what Alice felt like when she was falling down the hole into wonderland; I was Alice.

I am also following a mysterious rabbit that ends up bringing me on quite an adventure myself; Alice's mysterious white rabbit was my pain. I followed my pain down a huge hole just like Alice and her curiosity followed the rabbit. I was looking up, watching the sky get smaller and smaller as I fell farther and farther from the real world. I felt the thump that Alice felt when she got to the bottom of the hole, but for me it was the thump of my head against the kitchen floor after I passed out.

I had a choice, just like Alice, to drink from the bottle and to eat the cookie. I had a choice to give into my pain and follow it through the tiny door behind the curtain, to let it win, or to forget about it. I flooded the new world with my tears also, and floated with it downstream; where it was going, I didn't know.

Just like on her tears, I had no control of where I was going. Just like Alice, I met people I had never dreamed of meeting and did things that I never thought I would do.

Alice and I both fought for our sanity as we talked with people who weren't really there. We chased her rabbit and my pain down the path that the animated broom would automatically erase a couple of steps behind us; when we got lost and turned to see where we were, the path wasn't there anymore and we felt alone.

We had people tell us their strong opinions and what they thought we should do, but we also knew that they were wrong; she had the mad hatter and caterpillar, I had numerous doctors. She met the Queen of Hearts and had to battle her. Who's my Queen of Hearts? Is it Dr. Twenty-one? Am I going to have to battle her?

I hope not because even though Alice won, the Queen still decided that she lost. No matter how unfair it was, she was certain that Alice lost. Isn't that how everything goes? I can fight as hard as I want and for as long as I want, but it never pays off; someone or something will always come in and show me what I did wrong. I can never do anything and have it pay off; nothing I do is worth it. My fate will be decided, just like Alice's was, but unfortunately mine is not a dream that I can wake up from and have learned my lesson. Mine is real life, and there is no waking up from this.

Chapter Twenty-seven

"We are going to go into a forest today," Kathryn said calmly as she turned on soothing music. "Relax your body and feel yourself sink deeper and deeper into a peaceful place."

I lay back in the chair and let go of all my tension. I was extremely skeptical, but decided to give it all my effort and see where this went. *Couldn't hurt right?*

"Feel your bare feet gently step down onto grass and you see up ahead a big forest. You walk slowly towards it and make your way in through the huge trees. You walk through it, smelling all the pines around you and hearing the birds chirping, until you come to a small clearing. You hear some water and you follow the sound until you see a small pond…"

I was there; I could smell the pines, hear the birds, everything. I was suddenly in the forest behind my old house, the place that I was told my whole life not to go because there were coyotes, but now I was there and not scared at all. I was comfortable there, thanks to Kathryn.

While I was there I couldn't feel any pain. I wasn't thinking about school, and I wasn't worried about my parents. It was a place where I could just be with myself and enjoy it. In the forest I no longer resented myself for stealing away my youth or for keeping me up late at night crying. I was happy in the forest; for the first time in a long time I was genuinely content.

Maybe this stuff is going to work after all.

"Do you have any questions for Dr. Twenty-one?" my dad asked me in the UCLA waiting room.

"No," I replied. After about fifteen minutes they called me into the room where they took my temperature, blood pressure, weight, etc. and then to the room where I was to wait for Dr. Twenty-one.

No, not Dr. Twenty-one – Dr. Zeltzer. She was not just a number to me anymore, she was my doctor; Dr. Lonnie Zeltzer.

"Mommy, can you please rub my back?" It was really bothering me, so she came over and started to massage me.

Dr. Zeltzer came in and my mom moved back to her seat next to my dad. "Hey everyone," Dr. Zeltzer said smiling, "how are you all doing?"

"We are okay," my dad answered.

She looked at me. "Are you doing better, Georgia?"

"Sometimes," I said. "Some days I feel better and other days I feel worse than ever before."

"Let me give you a quick update," my dad spoke up; no matter what, there was always something to add to my journey. "She's still passing out, still running around and having those seizures. She has fallen a couple of times, saying she can't move, and she really can't for about an hour. Notre Dame asked us to remove Georgia from the school, so we did that a couple of days ago."

He continued, "But they did say that they were going to hold her spot for next year, so if she gets all her credits done by August, she can go back for her tenth grade year."

"Okay," Dr. Zeltzer said matter-of-factly, "then that's what we're gonna do."

I looked up at her. *How?*

"We are definitely going to get Georgia back for the tenth grade."

"How?" my mom asked.

"There are plenty of online correspondence courses available. You just have to contact the school and find out which ones they accept."

"I'll look into that," my dad volunteered.

"Okay," Dr. Zeltzer looked down at her clipboard, "now have we been reducing her doses on the medicine?" She was a lady on a mission.

"Just like you told us to…" The appointment went on just like any other doctor appointment would. She told me that at the last weekly meeting with the clinical team everyone who had worked with me had nice things to say about me.

"Now I have a question for you, but I don't want you to feel obligated to do this at all. There's a young woman, a graduate student at UCLA, who is studying anthropology. She is writing a research paper and has been using some of our students. Would you like to be part of it?"

"What do I have to do?" I asked.

"She follows you around with a video camera and comes to some of your appointments. If you don't feel comfortable with it, that's completely fine."

"I'll do it."

"Really?" she seemed surprised. "She's a very nice lady and if you're interested, I'll put you in contact with her."

"Okay, that'd be great," I said. I had no idea what this would entail, but I was willing to do anything; I just needed a purpose again. I wanted someone to tell my story.

"I have a question," my mom started. "What are we supposed to do about these seizures and her passing out?"

"I'm not too concerned by them," Dr. Zeltzer answered. *Not too concerned? What do I have to do to concern you; jump off a cliff?* "But if you would like some clarity, I can admit Georgia to the hospital and run some tests."

"What kind of tests?" I asked.

"They would measure your brain activity during a seizure versus when you aren't having one."

"Which hospital would we go to?" my dad asked.

"We can go to the one here at UCLA. Just tell me when you want to have this checked out," she said. "Personally, I think we should wait and see where things go."

"If it gets worse we'll call you," my dad said.

"Unless you have other questions, there is one more thing I would like to discuss before you leave," she looked right at me. "I would like you to get off the crutches."

Walking without the crutches proved to be a challenge; my leg was killing me and my back felt unsupported. I felt incomplete without my extra two feet since I'd been dependent on them for so long. While I was walking back to the car I kept whining and asking for my crutches, but my dad wouldn't budge. I knew I had to just push through it, but for some reason I couldn't. I was walking like a newly born colt when it first comes out of the womb, unstable and shaky.

I closed my eyes and pictured the pain on the floor and with each step I was defying it. I was stomping on it over and over again, imagining it getting smaller and smaller. But the pain wasn't diminishing; in fact, my stepping on the pain didn't do anything at all. I staggered all the way to the car, fighting back tears.

Admitted to the hospital? There is no way I am doing that. I am not going to stay overnight in one of those places; hell no. But at the same time, I did want answers. I did want to fix all these problems so I could live a normal, healthy life again. *Which one am I more scared of; sleeping overnight in a hospital bed or continuing to live in the unknown?*

"Hey there, Miss Georgia." I heard Phyllis sitting down next to me. I came out from under my covers and saw her figure in the darkness.

"What are you doing here?" I smiled.

"I just stopped by on my way back from work to see how you're doing," she said handing me a huge bouquet of assorted flowers.

I took them from her and smelled them. "Oh my gosh, what are these for?"

She shrugged, "Just to let you know we're all thinking about you."

"They're beautiful." My eyes started to tear up. "Thank you, Phyllis. Really."

The bouquet was filled with lots of different colors and types of flowers, but the one that really stood out to me was the sunflower. I see sunflowers as a symbol of hope. I admire the way they grow so tall because they can always find the sun. They reflect the sun's warmth with their yellow petals, like beams of sunshine. The true symbolic meaning of the sunflower is loyalty and dependability, which reflected my relationship with Phyllis. Along with others, Phyllis stood by me, through thick and thin, and was always there to offer her support. This whole pain thing was a true testament of my relationships with people.

"I thought today we could do some painting," Esther said, putting paintbrushes in front of me.

"I'm not good at painting," I said.

"You're going to be fine," she said, putting down a piece of paper for me to use.

Paint always made me nervous. I had so much more control with a pencil than with a paint brush. Also I had more freedom with a pencil because if I messed up I could just erase it; with paint, it was stuck there.

"I want you," she started, "to paint me a picture of what someone would see if they looked into your mind."

I thought about it for a while, feeling her eyes on my back. I picked up a paint brush and dipped it in the first color I saw. I continued painting, but in a careless manner. *If it's art therapy, I can do whatever I want.*

When I was done, she leaned it against the wall and we both stepped back to observe my work. It wasn't very pretty.

She studied it carefully. "Explain it to me."

"What do you mean?" She always asked such vague questions or made unclear statements. *Well, she is a shrink after all.*

"Tell me why you made it like this. Why would someone see your mind in this way?"

I looked at it and thought about it. "Well, I don't know if you can tell or not, but it's created as if someone is looking through a window into a house – like you wanted, a person looking into my mind. The curtain and the bars on the window are both dull, dismal colors. That signifies what someone notices when they look at me from the outside – they see me as nothing special. But, if you look inside the house you see the variety of bright, beautiful colors everywhere. If you were to look into my soul, or at least what it used to be, you would see a bright, beautiful, and confident girl who was happy. At first glance, someone wouldn't think much of me and my depressed exterior, but if they looked through the window, they would notice how great I really am."

"Have you told your parents how scared you are?" Beth asked as she adjusted my shoulders to properly mimic the pose. Even though she was the only person I was seeing who wasn't a therapist, I felt like I could be most honest with her.

"No, because they already have so much to deal with," I said, feeling the stretch in the back of my legs.

"But if it's really bothering you, you have to let them know."

"I'm sure they know that it scares me."

She thought about it for a second. "I think that if you're so concerned with your passing out, you should go to the hospital like Dr. Zeltzer suggested."

"But I don't want to go to the hospital," I whined.

"Would you rather have a rough night and peace of mind, or a night in your own bed, but tossing and turning?" *She has a point.*

I noticed a small yellow ball on the chair in the corner of grandpa's room. "What's this?" I asked picking it up.

He exclaimed, "Oh, thanks for reminding me!" Grandpa shot up, took it from my hands, and started into my grandma's room, "Follow me."

He called out to grandma, "Evelyn, Evelyn. The girls here are going to help us bowl."

"What?" Veronica and I laughed, looking at each other.

"What's this about?" my mom asked.

"I signed your mother up to go bowling next week," grandpa replied, "and she needs to practice. Georgia, you go over there and sit down. Veronica, you sit over there, and Lynn, you stay here with us." He directed and we obeyed.

My grandma used to love to bowl, that was her sport, but as she aged she stopped doing it. Now she was restricted to a wheelchair, but that didn't stop my grandpa; she was still the same, strong woman to him.

He wheeled her into the hallway and put the yellow ball in her hand. He held her hand and did the motions with her. Together they would roll the ball to me, the pretend pins. Then I would give the ball to my mom to run it back to them so they could do it again. After a while my grandma got the motion down and did some rolls herself.

That day showed me what unconditional love really was. All my grandpa wanted was to see my grandma happy doing something she used to love, because when the person you love is happy, you will be happy, too. Through thick and thin they had always been there for each other and after all these years they still loved each other so much.

"You have a message from that graduate student that Dr. Zeltzer talked to us about. You still want to do this?" my dad asked me one afternoon.

"Yes," I answered.

"Why?"

"I don't know, I just do." I really did know why I wanted to be a part of it. *If that's what she's studying, then she might be able to help me.*

Chapter Twenty-eight

"Dad!" I screamed. "Dad!"

He came running in. "What is it?"

I was on the floor in the dining room holding my head. "I think I really hurt myself." I closed my eyes and tried to calm down. *What was it that Kathryn told me?... I'm in a forest swimming with the fish in the stream? No, that's not right.*

"What were you doing in here?" he asked, confused.

"I wasn't," I started to see spots.

"Did you pass out and wake up here again?"

"I think so, but really dad, I hurt my head."

"Do you want to go to the ER?"

I took a deep breath, "I think it's time to do the tests."

We filled out the paperwork, we waited for hours; we talked to a nurse, and then waited for more hours. Even though I had an admittance request from a prestigious doctor from the hospital's university, I still didn't get great service, which surprised me. After six hours I was finally moved to a bed in the hallway; *not great, but progress.* That just goes to show you, it doesn't matter who you know or how you know them, you're just another whining problem to the ER staff.

A man with a clipboard took me out of the bed in the hallway and gave me my own room in the ER. I had my blood pressure and temperature taken by the nurse and even though I begged her not to, she put an IV in my arm. I didn't like her after that.

Okay, so now what? There was no TV. All I had was my chapstick.

"Oh my God, dad," my jaw dropped. "The iPhone is being delivered tomorrow, but we won't be home to sign for it."

"It's okay, just calm down. When are they coming?"

"In the middle of the day."

Noooo, I really wanted it.

"I'll try to have someone get it for you. It'll be okay, we'll get you your phone."

I didn't know what to do with my time. I wasn't used to having absolutely nothing to do. I'm the kind of person who needs to be busy every second of the day and when I didn't have anything to do, I felt like I was being tortured.

Slow down, you crazy child
you're so ambitious for a juvenile
But then if you're so smart, tell me
Why are you still so afraid?

Slow down, there is no other option for a patient in a hospital. I can only go at the pace of my doctors and nurses, which is not really fair or productive. *Crazy child*, yup... that's why I'm in this mess. I wouldn't call myself ambitious, more like desperate; desperate to find out what is really happening to me – and why. I am not smart, I am anything but that. I am as smart as I am happy. Do you really want to know the real reason I'm still afraid? Billy, I'm afraid of what they are going to say. Telling myself that I'm crazy is one thing, but hearing it from professionals would crush me. I'm scared they are going to confirm what I've been thinking all along.

"Can somebody help me?! Can somebody please help me?!"
Why is dad yelling?
I opened my eyes just in time to see two nurses run in and my sweating dad holding me down. I didn't need to ask, I knew what had happened.
"She's going to fall off the bed. Do you have straps or something?" my dad asked, clearly exhausted.
"I'm not going to be strapped down to the bed like a crazy person," I snapped.
"Something needs to hold you down. I can't do it. What if you fall?" he snapped back at me.
The nurse interrupted, "We can put up the sides of the bed."
"Yes," my dad relented, "please do that."

I was a baby in a crib; it was as simple as that. I used to put the barriers up on the beds of the little kids I would babysit. When they would ask me why they needed the barrier, I'd tell them that it was to keep them safe and to keep them from falling. I'd tell them that it was because I didn't want them to get hurt. Now I was the one being babysat and locked in. I was the one that no one wanted to get hurt. I was the one being protected from myself.

"Hey Georgia, it's Aunt Pam." Jenny's mom came into my room laughing.

"Aunt Pam?" I questioned.

She explained, "For me to get in here I needed to be immediate family."

"Oh, okay."

"Can you watch her while I make a phone call?" my dad asked.

"Yeah sure," she said sitting down.

"No, you need to be right next to her in case she has a seizure and then you have to literally hold her down."

Pam scooted her chair right up next to my crib and gave him a thumbs up, so he left.

"What are you doing here?" I asked.

"Can't I just come visit you?" she smiled.

"Yeah, I guess."

"How are you doing?"

"Bored out of my mind," I said, throwing the sheets off. I was getting hot.

She pulled her purse up onto her lap. "I figured that."

"What's in your bag?"

"I brought you stuff to do." She started pulling things out and putting them on top of me. "I brought you cards, a stress ball, chips, a sketch book, pencil…" *Pam, you are my hero.*

We played cards until my dad came back. Before Pam left she agreed to get my iPhone for me and bring it to the hospital the next day. A huge weight was lifted off my shoulders. I'd get my iPhone after all.

"If you need anything else, just buzz me," the nurse said after she took my blood pressure again.

"I have one question. Do you have any idea when I will be admitted into the hospital? Like in a real room?" I asked.

"No, I'm sorry, but this is a really busy day and they are completely packed up there." *Ugh.*

"Excuse me?" I called after a nurse walking by my room. "Do you know when I will be moved upstairs?"

"Sorry, I don't."

"Hey honey." My mom came in with a couple of bags.

"Hi Mommy," I smiled.

"How are you doing?" She sat down next to me.

"Not too well."

"Are you having pain?"

"It's really bad, mom." I put my head down.

"I'm so sorry," she hugged me. "I brought you some stuff. I brought you your toothbrush, asthma medicine, clothes...."

"Did you bring my iPod?" I interrupted.

She looked disappointed in herself. "No, I'm so sorry, honey. I didn't think to bring that." *Ugh.*

By the end of the night it was just my dad and me left, waiting. Every time we asked someone when I would be moved upstairs they said that they were extremely busy and that they didn't know.

Somebody just give me an answer already!

I fell asleep feeling really down. I was upset and all I wanted was to be as far away from the place as possible.

I hate hospitals.

It took them all night. They woke me up the next morning to tell me that I had a room – but of course we couldn't go up there because it wasn't ready. *Where did my dad sleep?* They were going to bring me up to my room as soon as possible.

We have a room! I was so happy. I called my mom and told her the news, which made her day.

We are on the way to figuring this out.

"Hi, my name's Tommy. Are you Georgia?" A young man came into my room.

"Yeah," I smiled. I was in a great mood and even though he was pulling a cart, he looked friendly so I wasn't nervous.

"How are you? I heard you got a room."

"Yeah I did. I'm doing a lot better now."

"Great," he nodded. "They're going to do tests on your brain when you go upstairs, so my job is to put the sensors on your head. That way they can hook up the wires to a machine and see your brain waves."

I started to get nervous. It felt like a sci-fi movie experiment. "Okay."

He began to pull out these wire things and bottle of a clear substance. He saw how nervous I was so he tried to comfort me. "I promise this doesn't hurt at all," he told me. "It looks scary but it's really not."

I trusted Tommy.

"Can you take your hair out of the bun please?"

"Yeah." When I did, he took the bottle and brought it to my head. I stopped him. "What's that?'

"It's glue."

Glue?! "Where's it gonna go?"

"On your head."

"In my hair?"

He understood and laughed. "Yes, most of it will be in your hair."

"What happens when we take it out? Will my hair come out, too?"

"No, I promise you it won't. I've done this many times. Your hair will be fine."

When he squirted the glue into my hair I felt like one of the ladies at the hair salon getting her roots touched up. He was putting glue at the very roots of my hair, as close to the skin as possible. The glue was cool and sticky, but it didn't bother me while he was putting it on.

After each glob of glue he placed a little metal cube into the glob and held it until it stuck. Later he attached the little wires to each metal cube and I was set. *I feel like a robot.*

"Okay Georgia," Tommy said while he was cleaning up his things. "They're going to hook you up to the machine once you get in your room. Do you have any questions?"

"Yeah, how do I get this stuff out of my hair afterward?"

He laughed, but I was serious. "You just wash your hair like you normally would and you'll be fine. Good luck, Georgia. It was nice meeting you."

"You too. Thanks."

A couple of hours went by of just waiting. *What happened to my room?*

My mom came to the hospital and when she walked in, she immediately froze. She was clearly surprised at something; *but what?*

She quickly composed herself. "Hey honey, how are you?"

"What's wrong?" I asked.

"Nothing," she gave me a fake smile.

"Why did you look like you saw a ghost?"

"Georgia, nothing's wrong," she said and pointed to my head. "What's all this?"

I knew it. "It's for when they look at my brain waves or whatever. Does it look that bad?"

She shook her head. "No, no. It doesn't look bad at all."

"Then why do you keep looking at it?"

"I'm sorry. I won't look anymore."

"I want to look."

"Are you sure?"

"Yes."

She searched through her purse and found her little pocket mirror. She opened it slowly, looked at it, and hesitantly handed it to me. I took it and looked in.

I'm a monster; I look like Medusa with her head of snakes. I had two metal blocks and wires on my forehead. The rest were spread out around my head. There were a lot of them and the glue stunk. *I look so scary.*

At lunchtime, they finally wheeled me up to my room. They had me change into a cloth hospital gown instead of a paper one. It was a much, much bigger room than my area downstairs and there were big windows. There were two beds in the room but one was empty. There were two TV's and my own personal bathroom. This was much better – except they had to put a new IV in my arm. I was officially admitted into the UCLA Hospital; *yay.*

I got up there just after they'd served lunch, so unfortunately I had to miss that meal for the day.

"Are you going to stay?" I asked my mom.

"Yes," she said squeezing my hand.

"Good," I smiled, "thanks."

Another doctor came in after about a half hour. "Hello, I'm Dr. Twenty-two. Are you Georgia Huston?"

"Yes."

"May I see your wristband?" I showed him the white hospital band around my wrist. New doctors always liked to see it; *like anyone would pretend to be me right now.* "Okay, great. So what's going on?"

"My husband explains it best. He's out in the hallway, let me go get him." My mom got up and stuck her head out the door to call my dad.

My dad came in and shook Dr. Twenty-two's hand, "Jimmy."

"Dr. Twenty-two," he responded. "I hear you're the man with the story."

"That would be me."

"Okay, so tell me why your daughter's here." *Here we go.*

He told about doctor after doctor, diagnosis after diagnosis. I totally zoned out, I knew it by heart. It felt like I had seen this movie too many times. I knew every line and what every actor did in each scene. I knew when he was going to make the jokes and when he was going to get serious. *I have to stop watching this movie.*

"I'm going to hook up the machine and then we will be all set. How does that sound?" Dr. Twenty-two asked smiling at me.

"Fabulous," I said sarcastically. *Dr. Twenty-two, be my hero.*

He had me sit up in my bed and put my head down a little. He wheeled over a machine and one by one attached each of the wires from my head to the wires from the machine. Dr. Twenty-two pressed a couple of buttons on the machine and left. He came back a few minutes later, wheeling in an even bigger machine.

He parked it right next to my bed. Dr. Twenty-two typed more things into that machine. He hooked my IV up to it and put a blood pressure cuff on me that was also connected to the bigger machine. *How do I move?*

"This machine," he said pointing, "is your IV. This cuff around your arm will be taking your blood pressure. The wires from your head will travel to this computer and show us your brain waves," he said, turning the monitor to me.

"Is that me?" I asked pointing to it. The girl on the screen pointed also.

"Yes, there is a camera watching you, so we can synch up what's happening in your brain with what's happening with your body." *I really am a science experiment.* "Any more questions?"

Yeah, when do I get out of here? "No, thank you," I politely smiled.

My mom went home to check on Veronica and my dad roamed the halls for most of the day. I was watching TV and randomly passing out and having seizures; *each one makes a difference!*

In the early evening, right after the cafeteria lady came to ask for my dinner order, my dad came in holding a small brown box.

"Pam just dropped this off for you." He handed it to me.

"My iPhone!" I ripped the box open.

"You need to call Pam and thank her because she had to chase down three different UPS trucks to find it."

"I will," I said, only half listening. When I took it out of the box I could hear the Hallelujah Chorus in the background; *my life is going to get better now.*

It turned out that I needed to install my phone through iTunes before I could really use it, so I still had to wait until I got home. I called Pam to thank her and then had dinner.

My mom, who seemed stressed, and Veronica, who seemed uncomfortable, arrived. We watched TV for a while, content and bored at the same time. I passed out and had another seizure.

I woke up exhausted, just as Dawn and Sarah made a surprise visit. Cheerful Dawn and hyper Sarah could always make me happy, and this time was no exception. Even though I couldn't really interact with them because of all the wires, it still made me really happy that they came.

Then our family friend Abe surprised me with a visit. He hung out with us for a while, too, which was so unexpected that I couldn't believe it. He was probably the last person that I would expect to show up, but he was the only person to come who wasn't family. That just proved again how sometimes it was the most unanticipated people who would make the biggest difference. People went out of their way to make me smile when they didn't have to do anything at all.

They all went home when visiting hours were over, but I will never forget them coming to visit me that evening. My dad offered to stay with me overnight, but my mom differed. She told him to go home and get some rest. So, my dad went home with Veronica while my mom slept over with me in the hospital.

"Mom, you don't have to stay here. I'm fine, really. There's nothing you can do," I told her over and over again, but secretly I really wanted her to stay.

"No, Ms. Peaches, just try to get some sleep," she shooed me away.

"Where are you going to sleep?"

"Right here," she put her arms out jokingly and smiled.

"You are not sleeping in a chair," I scolded her.

"Yes I am."

"No, you're not. Come into my bed," I said scooting over.

"No, that's your bed. We won't fit comfortably."

"I'd rather us both be a little uncomfortable than you be completely uncomfortable."

"George, I'm fine."

"Please mom, just come into bed."

We cuddled all night together in a hospital bed that could barely fit one comfortably. She stayed there with me even though I was hogging all the blankets, walked me back and forth to the bathroom with my machines, and held me down during seizures. She was there for me that night, all night, for whatever I needed. It made a big difference having her there next to me.

Everyone who has spent a night in a hospital knows that it is impossible to have a good night's sleep; and that was my second night there, so I was really behind on my sleep. I couldn't get any sleep because – besides the fact that the beds are uncomfortable and it's always freezing – people are constantly bothering you. They are taking your blood pressure, checking your IV; they seem to visit you more at night when you're trying to sleep than during the day when you actually need them.

When we woke up, my dad was already sitting in the room with us. They brought me an awful breakfast that I didn't eat, but I usually don't have breakfast anyway. The nurses kept coming in and telling us that the doctor was going to be right in, and then they would come back an hour later and tell us the same thing. It was extremely frustrating; *but where's the surprise there?*

My dad left the room for a little bit and when he came back, he wasn't just with one doctor; he was with a group of white lab coats.

"Hello Georgia," the oldest doctor shook my hand. "I'm Dr. Twenty-three." *Dr. Twenty-three, be my hero.*

"Hi," I smiled. None of the other lab coats introduced themselves, but they were Doctors Twenty-four through Twenty-nine. They were all neurologists.

"We have looked at the tests," my heart was following his every word, "and we don't see any reason for you to be having these 'seizures.'" He put his hands up and mockingly quoted the word "seizure."

"So then what is it?" I asked. My dad was standing behind them listening, but not reacting; they had already told him everything, so none of this was a surprise.

"I think you are having what we call 'pseudo-seizures.'" *What?!*

"'Pseudo?'" I asked pathetically, "Like fake?"

"Not fake, exactly," he seemed to be choosing his words very carefully. "We think of it in terms of 'self-proclaimed' seizures."

"Like I'm making them up?" I could feel my face getting red.

"We don't know what's going on," he dodged the question.

"Well, who would know?" I was getting mad. "You were supposed to have the answers," I accused him.

"The tests don't show any significant change in your brain waves, so we don't know exactly." *Stop BSing me!*

I closed my eyes and took a deep breath; *am I really ready for the answer to my next question?*

"Am I crazy?"

In the background, I could see my dad's body straighten. He looked on edge.

"We don't know what's going on," the doctor repeated. *Stop saying that and just give me an answer!*

"Am I crazy?" I asked again.

"What does crazy really mean?"

Chapter Twenty-nine

I plopped down in my own bed, sobbing. My parents sat next to me so I threw the blanket over me, even though it was really hot.

"Oh George, come on," my mom tried to pull the blanket off, but I didn't loosen my grip.

"Georgia, we need to talk to you," my dad said calmly.

"Go away! Everyone leave me alone," I pleaded.

"Peaches...."

"Please," I interrupted.

Nobody spoke for a moment. "Georgia," my dad started, "we need to talk."

I threw up the covers, "What?! What do you need to talk to me about, huh? Do you want to know why I'm making all this up, too? Do you want to know why I'm putting you guys through this? Do you want to know how much fun it is?!"

"Georgia, you are not making this up," my dad put his hand on my shoulder.

"Yes I am! Are you not listening to all these doctors? Well unfortunately, I am. I'm hanging on every fucking word!"

My mom cringed at my crude language and I had never seen such a distressed look on my dad's face before. "Please Georgia," he begged. "Listen to me. You are not making this up."

"Stop telling me what I'm doing! Don't you think I would know a little better than you?"

"What makes you think that?" my mom asked. "Just because they can't see it doesn't mean that it's all in your head."

"How are you going to sit there and tell me that? How are you going to lie to me?!"

"Georgia, this is real. There is a real reason that all this is going on," my dad said. "You have chronic pain, you need to realize that. You need to realize that it's not you."

"Then who is it? It's all in my head, I'm the one that is making this up," I said through my tears. "I'm the crazy one."

"You're not crazy," my mom hugged me; her cheeks were wet.

"I am! I don't know how many stupid doctors we have to go to for you guys to get that through your heads, but when they're all telling me that, what do you expect me to think?!"

"No doctor has ever told you that you were crazy," my dad said.

"No?" I challenged him, "You were in the fricken room!"

"He didn't say...."

"No, listen to me," I ordered. "I asked him straight up if I was crazy. What was his answer? Do either of you remember?"

"He said 'no,'" my dad said.

"No! He didn't say 'no!'"

"Then what did he say?" my mom asked.

"He never said 'no.' He dodged that question like it was the plague. He just found other ways to answer it in a politically correct way. You tell me, explain to me please, how I'm supposed to take it when one of the highest regarded individuals in this field won't simply answer 'no' to such a defining and important question. Tell me!" I'd never let so much out with so much anger in my whole life.

My parents looked at each other and I could tell I stumped both of them. "He didn't say you were crazy," my mom mumbled.

"But he didn't say I wasn't."

"You see all your problems, everyone that makes you uncomfortable or doubt yourself. Visualize them in your mind... Then, like a camera zooming back from a scene, zoom away from them... As you back up, you notice that they have been standing behind a window... You watch the window close as you continue to zoom out and away from their negative attitudes... The curtain closes and it starts to rain; it's raining so hard that you can only see the outline of their bodies through the curtain... You zoom out farther and you watch them turn and walk away. You realize that it's not you, it's them. They are the problem and now they are out of your life... You feel relieved as you notice your negative energy being flushed out of your body. You feel happy because now there is no more bad in your life." Kathryn was doing her best to get me in a better place.

I was always impressed after my appointments with Kathryn. I never left there feeling the same as when I went in; I was always better. I needed hypnotherapy; I needed Kathryn.

"How am I supposed to do an art piece with tape?" I was very confused.

"Look," Esther pointed to the bucket in front of me filled with different sizes of tape and in every color imaginable. "Just put the tape on the paper however you want."

I had never in my life even considered using tape to draw, but whatever; she's the expert. It took me a while to do it since I wasn't used to that medium, but as soon as I was done, she leaned it against the wall like usual.

"How was it using the tape?" she asked.

"It took me a while to get used to it," I said looking at my "art."

"Well I must say, you really figured it out," she seemed genuinely impressed. "Tell me about it."

"I know it's depressing." I was a little disappointed with how sad it looked; it was full of resentment. "The dark blue tape makes a corner, do you see there? Then the light blue tape, I don't know if you can see it or not, but it's supposed to be a person sitting in the corner. The knees are up, the arms are crossed, and the head is down in the arms; I know it's hard to see but it's supposed to illustrate a very sad position. The body language shows distress, pain and suffering."

"The green ribbon in the corner shows how envious I am. All I have seemed to want in the past year is everything that I can't have, but think I deserve."

"As you can see, the pink tape says "LIES," a recurring theme in my art. I feel like I am constantly being lied to or treated like a baby. I know I'm not an adult, and I'm not trying to be, but I hate when the doctors talk to my parents behind my back. I'm not paranoid. I know what they tell them. The doctors say that I'm faking – my parents confided that to me."

"Nobody believes me or even respects me enough to tell me up front. I can deal with the truth and I deserve to feel respected by the phony doctors who look down on me like a whiney brat who just wants attention. That's what this tape 'art' is all about."

Esther sat there for a moment, soaking it all in. "Well if you want to stop the lies, then why don't you start showing the truth? Show them what's actually going on."

"How?"

"Don't let them win – and most of all – don't let chronic pain win."

"You act like it's a battle."

She shook her head. "It's not a battle, it's a war. It has been going on for way too long and I know how sick of it you are, and since I know you don't like lies, I'm going to tell you the truth. Chronic pain is a huge struggle, I know, and one that I'm not sure will have a definite ending. I know that's not what you want to hear, but some people never have a life without it."

I put my head down.

Esther continued, "I'm not telling you this to depress you, so look up at me. I'm telling you this to wake you up. I'm telling you this to inspire you. You are such a strong woman, and once you realize your full potential, this pain will never be a problem for you again. The only one who can stop this and help yourself is you. We can talk to you and give you all the tips in the world, but it's up to you to put all this training into action. You need to work on this if you want to get rid of it."

My dad opened the front door, "She's here." In walked a young lady with dark hair and glasses.

"Hi," she smiled. "I'm Mira."

"I'm Georgia," I said.

I introduced her to my parents and we all sat down.

Mira started, "So did Dr. Zeltzer explain to you what I'm doing?"

"A little bit, but not in much detail," my mom answered.

"Well, I am a graduate student in anthropology and for my research I'm studying the effects of pain on children," she explained. "I'm following a couple of other families and I would love to follow Georgia's journey as well."

"What would that entail?" my mom asked; I could tell she was very uncomfortable with this.

"Ideally Georgia would take a video camera, I will provide it, and do a kind of video diary. No one will see those videos but me, and I will just be using them for research; I promise no one else will see them. I would like to accompany you guys to doctors' appointments and if possible film those as well. I have 'Target' gift cards supplied by my grant to give your family if you are interested."

"Like a documentary?" I asked.

"No, I'm just using the film to observe and record for my paper."

"What do you think, Georgia?" my dad asked.

I thought a moment, "I want to do it."

"Great," she smiled, "are you two comfortable with it?"

"I am," my dad said. All heads turned to my mom. "Lynn?"

She didn't say anything at first, and then her first words were not very encouraging. "I don't know."

"If you don't feel comfortable with everything, you can tell me what you are okay with doing. This is all about you guys and I will never invade your privacy," Mira explained.

"Mom," I insisted, "I want to do it."

"Can we talk about this?" she asked my dad and me.

"No mom, I'm doing this," I respectfully answered. "This is my thing."

My mom did not seem happy, but finally agreed. "Fine."

"Are you sure?" Mira asked all of us.

"Yes," I smiled.

"Great, I'm very excited." Mira seemed to light up. "I have some paperwork for you to fill out." She handed us some packets that we started filling out.

"Let me give you some background on Georgia and tell you what's going on," my dad said; *ugh*.

We all filled out our papers and she gave me my own video camera. "How often do you want me to do this?"

She thought about it. "Whenever you can. Every night would be ideal, but I understand if you can't."

"What do you want me to say to it?"

"Anything you want, I just want you to keep me up to date on what's going on and what you're feeling. Here is a packet of questions to get you going if you can't think of anything, but I will be beyond happy with anything you give me."

"Do we tell you when her appointments are?" my dad asked.

"No, Dr. Zeltzer's office will do that. I'll just see you there."

"How often will I see you?" I asked.

"I don't want to be a bother, so it won't be too often, but I want you to call me if you have any questions or need anything. If you need a ride somewhere or just want someone to talk to, I'm here. I really want you to know that," she offered.

I smiled, "Great, thanks." *I barely know you; I doubt we are going to get close.*

I sat in bed and stared at the video camera; *now what?* I turned on the lamp next to my bed, ruining the darkness, and pressed the red button.

RECORD:

"Hi, it's umm Tuesday. Today we met and talked a little. I'm excited to do this study even though I don't really understand what it's for. When you left, my mom was really mad at my dad and me. She does not want us to do this at all and I don't really know why. It's nothing against you – she's just weird like that." *Who was I talking to, the camera or Mira?*

"I don't know how many other kids you are doing this with, or what they are going through, but I have really been through a lot. My dad told you most of it, but he didn't really explain to you the psychological traumas that I have been experiencing."

"Everyone keeps saying that I have chronic pain, but no matter how many times they explain it to me I cannot, for the life of me, wrap my head around it. They tell me that it has something to do with the receptors in my brain, not my back or leg, but then they tell me that I'm not crazy. Do they not understand that having something wrong with my brain and being crazy is the same thing?"

"Nobody understands what I've gone through. I have lost everything. I've lost my friends, my social life, my self-esteem, my mind – everything. I'm a loser who is making everyone else's life miserable, but the thing is, no matter how hard I try to stop it, I can't."

"If there is no reason for the pain, then why can't I stop it? That is my biggest struggle right now, trying to figure out why a pain that's not there can impact my life so much. Dr. Zeltzer says there are other kids out there going through everything that I'm experiencing, but how many kids could there possibly be? I've never heard of this. If what she says is true and other kids have this, then why don't more people know about it?"

"What if she just made this thing up to make me feel less alone? That's my main feeling – feeling alone. I think that's why I agreed to do this whole study thing with you – hearing that someone was actually interested in what's going on and wants to bring to light what I am going through got my interest. I want people to hear and know what I have been through."

"I want to make sure no one has to go through this again. I want to be given a voice because I deserve a voice. Everyone deserves a voice."

We needed money. All the therapies I was doing were coming straight out of our pockets; insurances didn't recognize them as medical therapies so we were on our own.

My parents used to be amateur race car drivers and my dad's favorite car was a vintage Lotus Elan. He loved that car so much; he'd completely restored it himself. When people thought of him in those days, they thought of that car – it was a part of him – but we needed the money.

Our close family friends in Texas, Andy and Terri, agreed to buy it. They were racing buddies of my parents and Andy still restored cars; but really they were just helping us out.

I needed to get out of town anyway, so I decided I was going to go with my dad to deliver the car. I needed a little change of scenery. *To Texas!*

The Lotus had been disassembled into a zillion pieces, so somehow we managed to fit the whole car, my dad's first baby, into our van. It wasn't easy, but we did it. We drove without stopping through California, Arizona, New Mexico, and half of Texas.

At one point I started having really bad back pain, so we stopped at a truck stop in the middle of nowhere. I took out my yoga mat and did yoga on the side of the empty highway. It really helped, but I was much happier when we finally got to Fort Worth.

I had always loved Andy and Terri. They were funky artists and college art teachers and just overall really fun and caring people. We visited them every summer; *I guess this one isn't an exception.*

When we pulled up, Andy had a few of his students help unload the van. I could see how down my dad was as they moved the pieces of his car into Andy's shop. He knew that it was the right thing to do, but it was still hard. We had all been giving up a lot lately.

We only stayed for a couple of days, but those days were awesome. Whenever I visited, Terri always gave me art assignments and we would do them together. This time she got us boxes that we were going to make into books somehow. She called them "book boxes" and it didn't really make sense but it ended up looking really cool. I made one for my mom and I was really proud of it. It was full of happy pictures and words of encouragement.

Terri drove a beautiful new Mini-Cooper convertible, which just happened to be my dream car. When I mentioned that to her she insisted that we go out driving that afternoon. I thought she was kidding but she wasn't; she said all I had to do was get it cleared by both my parents.

I thought there was no way that they would ever agree, but they both did – even though it was illegal since I was barely fifteen.

We found a large parking lot and I nervously switched seats with Terri. I looked down and to my horror I noticed that it was a stick shift – *I can't even drive an automatic.*

"I can't do this, Terri," I said looking at her.

"Oh come on," she playfully slapped my arm, "of course you can."

She talked me through it and before I knew it, I was driving a stick shift. It was only an empty parking lot in the middle of Texas – but I was driving! *Me; the girl who couldn't shower by herself.*

I couldn't believe it. I was on top of the world. Terri's faith and confidence inspired me to have faith and confidence in myself. That hour or two of her sitting in the passenger seat and trusting me with her prized car, the fact that she believed in me that much, made such a difference in the way I thought of myself.

Chapter Thirty

I was getting a call from an unknown number. "Hello?"

"Hi, is this Georgia?" a preppy voice on the other side asked.

"Yeah..."

"Hey! It's Bailey from Notre Dame."

Who? "Oh, hey Bailey. How are you?" I had literally no idea who this girl was.

"I'm great. How are you?"

"Oh, I've been better."

"I got your number from Raquel. I hope you don't mind."

"Not at all, what's up?"

"I didn't want to bother you, but I just wanted to call and let you know that everyone is thinking about you and praying for you."

I started to tear up. "Really?"

"Yeah," she said, "I'm not calling to interrogate you or to get the gossip, I just wanted to let you know that we are all rooting for you."

"Thank you so much."

"I mean it though, we are all here for you." Neither of us said anything for a second. "I'll let you go, but if you need anything at all, please just call me. Okay?"

"Okay, thank you so much, Bailey. You have no idea how much your call just meant to me."

"I'm glad. Come back to school, okay?"

"Okay."

After I hung up I racked my brain, trying to figure out who this Bailey girl was. Finally I remembered that she was a random girl in my first semester gym class who I'd barely talked to.

Wow. That is one incredible person. That one call that she probably doesn't even remember making was the turning point in my life; I will never forget that little conversation.

But you know that when the truth is told...
That you can get what you want or you can just get old
You're gonna kick off before you even
Get halfway through
When will you realize, Vienna waits for you?

Sometimes the truth isn't "told" to you; sometimes you have to find it for yourself. We feel like we deserve the truth, but it's not that easy. Truth is not given, it is earned. I have to earn my own truths. I am going to get what I want; no more lying in bed wishing for it. I'm kicking off right now, not the way I did before; not with a downward kick. This time I'm going up. Vienna, I'm coming, even if it kills me.

I pressed the button and took a deep breath.

> RECORD:
> "Hi. This is Wednesday and today something really amazing happened. This girl from school called me, and I didn't even know who she was at first, but she called just to let me know that she was thinking about me. I figured out who she was afterwards, but oh my God, I get emotional just thinking about it."
>
> "She asked me to come back to school, and I told her I would. Notre Dame's holding my spot, and I am going to fill it next fall. Dr. Zeltzer has told me over and over again how I need to stop feeling sorry for myself and get out of bed. Well she's right. It's up to me to get better and the sooner I get that through my head, the sooner I will be better."

I pressed PAUSE for a moment and laid down, focusing the camera back onto my face.

> RECORD:
> "I'm going to get better."

I got up and looked at a figure in my full-length mirror. I looked at her posture and her messy hair; I looked at her clenched jaw and her determined eyes. I turned around and went to my desk. I took out a green

Sharpie and went over to my mirror. I took the cap off the marker and wrote in the upper right hand corner, "7/11."

I wrote the date. I wrote the day that I stopped passing out.

In the morning I told my dad the news.

"I'm not going to pass out anymore."

"What do you mean?" he asked.

"I'm done being sick."

"I don't get it."

"I have goals. I thought them up last night. I want to be normal so I have a few favors to ask you for. Can you call Notre Dame and ask what courses they accept, like Dr. Zeltzer said to do? I am going to go back to school this fall," I promised. "Also, I wrote down the date of yesterday, my last day passing out, so in a couple of months, when I haven't passed out since '7/11,' I would like you to take me to get my driving permit test. I will be able to get it in November, so if I don't pass out until then, I want to learn how to drive."

"I'll see what I can do." My dad seemed pleasantly surprised and when I left the room I heard him chuckle.

"…then you put your legs up on the wall and walk your hands down your back, like this. Then you are in a shoulder stand." Beth showed me and then slowly got out.

"I can't do that," I said, nervously eyeing Mira in the corner of the room. She was observing my yoga class.

"Yes, you can. Come on. Put your butt against the wall and then whip your legs across and up the wall like I did. There you go, now push off the wall and hold your back with your arms. That's right, straight legs, I'm here to catch you if you fall." She was right next to me with her arms outstretched. Then she smiled, "You're doing it."

I was doing the shoulder stand, the pose that seemed so impossible to do. I was holding myself up with my shoulders, upside down; I was defying gravity. I will never forget that feeling, which I couldn't have gotten without Beth's support and encouragement.

"Sorry, I just got off the phone with my dad," I said after the appointment. "He said he's going to be a little late. Is that okay?"

"Yes," Beth said, "of course."

"I can take you home," Mira offered.

"Oh no, it's fine, but thank you," I politely declined.

"Georgia, it's no trouble. You guys are really helping me out, It's the least I can do. Will you call him and ask if it would help?"

Mira drove me home that day, which I expected to feel extremely guilty about. I hated being a bother for people, but Mira didn't make me feel that way at all. We talked and laughed with each other as we drove through the canyon. She was really nice and I enjoyed spending time with her.

"I spoke to Notre Dame today," my dad reported. "They said that if you want to come back next fall you have to have all your credits done by early August."

"How am I supposed to do a semester's worth of work in barely two months?" I asked.

"We can do it," he said. "I'll order your courses today."

I woke up in the middle of the night feeling the familiar excruciating pain in my back. I grabbed my back, wincing; I looked around to see if my parents were awake. Nope, I was the only one awake in the house. *Now what?*

Someone is stabbing my back, but why? Why are they doing this to me? I was just getting over this; I was just beginning to fight back. Is this what Dr. Zeltzer was talking about? Okay, try to remember what she told me.

I took a deep breath and closed my eyes.

She told me that the pain won't necessarily stop coming, but it's up to me to decide how long it will stay. She said that I need to stop feeling sorry for myself and I need to continue on with my life. She told me that I needed to use my tools.

My tools... I can't do craniosacral massage, that's something I need Chris for. Chris is coming this afternoon, why couldn't he be here now? Okay, he's not here; so now what?

My back was killing me; *I don't think I can do this.*

Yes I can. Remember the "7/11" on my mirror? That was a promise I made to everyone. I made for my parents, for Veronica, and for myself. I always keep my promises. "7/11" is the last day that I am going to pass out. It was the last day of my old life. My new life starts now.

I can't do art therapy, it's too dark and I don't want to wake anyone else by walking around. If I do yoga that means that I would have to get out of bed, also waking my parents. I couldn't wake them up; they have been working too hard. They deserve a good night's sleep; they deserve a break. Hypnotherapy, I can use my hypnotherapy... But how?

Our hypnotherapies seem to change for every appointment so there's no way for me to really copy it.

The pain was blinding me and my thoughts; my breath was getting faster and I could feel a panic attack coming on; *no, this cannot happen. I won't let this happen.*

As I felt myself slowly losing my mind and letting the panic attack win, I tried to think about another place that I could go. I tried to imagine going back to the forest like when I went with Kathryn, but for some reason I couldn't picture the trees or hear the stream. My heart sank as I realized that I was on my own. I took deep breaths and sank deep into a relaxed state; *my mind will take me to where I should go.*

With my eyes closed I could feel a breeze on my face and my bare feet. My hands were buried deep into sand and when I opened my eyes I could see where I was.

I was at the beach.

I could hear the ocean, but I couldn't really see it yet. I was at the same beach as the beach house, but I wasn't there.

Instead, just down the beach are some sand dunes that I always loved going to; that's where I was right now. I looked around and the beach was empty; I was all alone. But, for some reason that didn't scare me, it made me feel safer.

I stood up and slowly walked up the sand dune. Usually it was hard to walk up the dune because I would sink in the sand, so it took a lot of effort. But, this time it wasn't like that. This time I could just walk on the surface like it was normal ground; I was no longer sinking. When I got to the top of the dune the wind hit my face; I made it. I looked out to the water and saw the sun setting. It wasn't too cold or too hot; it was perfect.

Is this my Vienna? Did I finally make it?

I feel like that night was crucial to defeating my pain. It was a test, and I won. For the first time, I felt like I had the power; I could control my own life. At first I thought I might be getting ahead of myself by thinking I was going to get better – but why not? What's stopping me?

I smiled; *I'm going to keep my promise.*

Chapter Thirty-one

Chris came over, as scheduled, and gave me the massage of my life. He always blew me away by how little he would touch me, but what a big impact it would make. My dad always jokes that every time he came through the room it looked like Chris was in the same exact position, which was true. It didn't seem like he ever moved.

He always made me happy, too, just by his manner. He had a way of relaxing me, even by just having a conversation. The smell of lavender always makes me think of him because that's the smell that always followed when I saw him.

My dad and I drove past Notre Dame on the way to pick up Veronica at her school. It was very bittersweet as I passed the campus that was once my home. I thought back to when I was a student there. I remembered walking in the halls and around the quad, thinking that this was all there was to life. It was an unexplored concept for me that life went on beyond the gates. We all went into school at seven forty-five and left at three, but while we were in school, other people weren't part of our universe.

Cars were still driving, restaurants were still open, and kids were still playing at parks. It seemed so odd to me that there was a world outside of mine. Life went on, even when I wasn't there to go on with it.

Now it was the opposite. Now I was on the outside in the real world and all I wanted to do was go through those gates and slip back into my desk like nothing happened. Now I was in the real world and I didn't want any part of it, I didn't care that cars were still driving down the streets, I wanted to gossip at lunch and take tests that I didn't study for. I was on the outside, and I didn't like it at all; *life out here sucks.*

I turned on Mira's video camera. I always started recording before I figured out what I was going to say.

RECORD:

"It's umm Thursday. Today was all right. I had yoga with Beth and that was pretty much it."

"Whenever I go to Beth's or Kathryn's or Esther's we have to drive through this street called Beverly Glen. I don't know why, but I really like that street and it immediately relaxes me."

"I don't know if it's because I associate the street with all the relaxing therapies I do right after it, or if the street's just magic, but for some reason I really like that street. You're the anthropology person, you tell me! I like the shade and I like how all the houses are really close, almost on top of each other. It cuts through a canyon, which is pretty cool because it's this really small and winding road. When we drive through it I feel like I'm driving through a backyard or something because everything is so tight."

"I would never want to live there, but for some reason that street just attracts me. There's a park that's really pretty, but it's usually empty. When it's not, there are only a few kids there with their nannies; I don't know if it's because of the time of day we go or if it's just not a popular park, but I really like it."

"I decided today that when I'm all better and back at Notre Dame with my friends, I am going to go to that park to celebrate. I really want to go to that park, so when I'm all better, I will."

I didn't pass out all day! — (knock on wood...)
My dad came in the living room where I was sitting on the couch.
"Hey, I signed you up for your courses."
My heart skipped a beat. "Really? Okay, what do I do now?"
"They're going to send you the papers and everything. They will probably get here in a couple of days. But, you've started the process."
"Okay, good. Thanks."

I wanted to play some games online, so I turned on my mom's laptop and waited for everything to load. As I was sitting at her work area, naturally my eyes started to wander around the table at all her papers.

I didn't touch any at first, but my eyes caught one that I felt compelled to look at; it was from a hospital. I tried to read it, but didn't really understand what it was saying. All I could get from it was that my mom had some tests done. I wasn't really concerned; *don't adults have to get check-ups after a certain age?* She was my mom, she was fine. I continued to play games, trying to pass the time until my school courses came in the mail, whenever that would be.

"I'm going to take you to Esther's today," my mom said smiling.
I was happy. "Really? Cool, you'll really like her."
"I'm gonna take you to Beth's after, too."
"Awesome," I smiled. "Let's go."

"Hi, Esther," I said proudly when she opened the door. "This is my mom."
"Oh, hi. How are you? It's so nice to meet you," she said shaking my mom's hand.
"Thanks, you too," my mom smiled.
"Are you going to wait here or go out during the appointment?" Esther asked.
"I don't know. What do you suggest?"
I'd forgotten to mention to my mom that she was going to be on her own for an hour.
"There are a lot of shops downstairs you can look at," I said.
"Okay, I'll do that," my mom said, waving and walking out the door. "I'll see you in an hour."
Esther and I got settled in. I was at the desk and she was next to me in her chair. "You look just like your mother," she said laughing.
"I know," I said smiling, "everyone always says that."

"So tell me about this. What does it represent?" Esther asked when I was done and leaned it against the wall.
I looked at my empty picture, wondering if I should have put more on the page; *no, it's perfect.*
"Well, I drew the man on the left side of the page in gray because gray represents the gloominess and hopelessness that I've been feeling. The reason he is so crudely done with such harsh lines is that everyone is a little rough around the edges. The red balloon in the middle of the page symbolizes happiness and joy. The figure is holding the balloon trailing behind. Even though he is turned away and might not see it

at the time, it's there. There is always something good that's going to come, and as long as he turns to see it and is open to it, he will start living his life on his own terms."

Esther nodded a couple of times, digesting what I said, and then asked, "Are you living your life on your own terms?"

"No."

"Why not?"

"Because I can't," I complained.

"What's stopping you?"

"My pain."

"Who's stopping you?"

I was confused. "Stopping me from what?"

"From living a life without pain," she explained.

I thought about it. "Me, I guess."

"So now what do we do?" my mom asked when we got in the car. It was fun how new to this she was, since she was usually working.

"We have a couple of hours to kill. Do you want to go to lunch?" I suggested. It didn't make sense to go all the way home.

"That sounds good."

We went to lunch together and it was really fun because we hadn't been spending a lot of time together, just the two of us, and when we were, it was always about my health problems.

After lunch we went shopping in Beverly Hills, even though we knew we weren't going to buy anything, but sometimes that's the best kind of shopping. I always loved fooling around while shopping. Sometimes I would grab the most ridiculous clothes I could find in the store and try them on just for the heck of it.

I introduced her to Beth, who she loved, and she watched my yoga lesson. I loved having her there because I thought that I had gotten pretty good at yoga and I wanted to show her how hard it was, but that I could do it. I was really proud to show her all the things that I had been doing and to give faces to some of the people that I had been talking about so much lately. That day always stood out to me because it was just my mom and me and I was really missing those days.

On the way back home from that fun day I was staring out the window and my mind was wandering.

"Hey mom?" I asked, "what was that test you did at the hospital for?"

She looked very surprised, "What are you talking about?"

"I saw it on your desk when I was on your computer yesterday," I said embarrassed. *I shouldn't have brought this up.*

"Oh, that was just a checkup thing," she said shortly.

"For what?" I pressed.

"They were checking for something, but I got the results and everything's okay," she seemed to desperately want to get off the topic, but that just made me want to get to the bottom of it even more.

"Promise?" I respected her wishes.

"I promise, baby." She gave me a reassuring smile.

Chapter Thirty-two

My dad came in holding a big fat envelope and threw it down on the bed next to me, smiling.

"What's this?" I asked, picking it up.

"Your courses. You can start today."

Oh my gosh, finally! School starts at the end of August. I'm already so far behind. Time's running out, but I can do it.

I opened the envelope and flipped through the course books. "Which one should I start with?" I asked my dad.

"What do you think will be easiest?"

"I don't know, world geography?"

"Okay then," he nodded, "start with that."

I opened it up and there was a note from my "teacher." She wasn't really my teacher. She was just the one who made the course. She wrote about her background and how to do well in this course, etc. There was even a little picture of her. I skimmed it, but that's it.

Honestly, I didn't do much work for my world geography class. I knew most of it already. A lot of it was just terms that anyone with common sense would know and when it came to geography, I had been to every continental state in the United States, so I knew my way around the U.S.

At the end of each lesson there was a little ten question quiz that I had to do and then log onto my account on the computer and input my answers. They were instantly corrected, so I knew right away what my grade was, which was nice. If I didn't pass the quiz, then I had one more try to retake it, but I never had to retake any for world geography. I got through that course in two days, *piece of cake*. I was feeling extremely optimistic about getting all of this done in time.

When I was finished with that course's work, I had to take a final exam. It had to be proctored by a certified person, and luckily an administrator at Notre Dame was qualified and willing – Mr. Klee graciously agreed to proctor my exam. I was to go to his office a couple of days later to take it. I had scheduled it after school on purpose, in an attempt to prevent seeing anyone from my classes. I wasn't ready yet.

"Where are your crutches?" Sarah asked when I hugged her.
"I don't have them anymore," I said proudly.
"Why not?" She seemed confused.
"Because I'm all better now," I lied. *Do white lies count as lies?*
"Do you sleep here?" Sarah was talking about the mattresses on the floor of the living room.
I hugged Dawn and Steve, who'd just arrived. "Yes I do, baby."
"Why?"
"I like to keep the doggies company at night." That made her laugh.
"Where are your parents?" Dawn asked.
"Picking up grandpa," I replied, sitting down on the couch next to Steve.
"Is Veronica still at school?"
"Yeah, she just stayed there after school."
"Is she excited?"
"I think so."
Veronica was in her school musical, "Into the Woods." She had been going to rehearsals every day after school and practicing at home. She had been in the chorus throughout elementary school, but this was her first full-length production and we were all going to be there to see it.
I thought about how it was her night and I hoped that my health problems wouldn't get in the way of it. 7/11... 7/11... Whenever I started to feel anxious I would think that to remind myself of my promise – of my goal.
I sat in between my grandpa and Sarah, who was dressed up like a fairy. Talia was in the same play at her high school a couple of years before that and Sarah loved the fairies in it. That was why she had a fairy skirt on; she was in costume.
It was a middle school production so we weren't expecting a lot, but it was actually pretty good. Veronica didn't have a big part but when she was on stage, she shined. After the play she came running out with her friends in her costume and make-up, absolutely glowing. We gave her flowers and she seemed like she was on top of the world; everything was about her for that night and I was happy for her.

I turned the camera toward me, hair up and bags under my eyes.

RECORD:

"Today was Veronica's school play. It was okay, but it made me think back to my "Joseph and the Amazing Technicolor Dreamcoat" days in Hollywood. It reminded me of how proud I was coming off that stage, knowing that people paid to watch me perform. I knew it wasn't just me and that I only had a small part, but at least I was part of it. I remember not wanting to take off my costume or make-up because that meant the performance was over; that I was normal again and no one was watching me anymore."

"I think it's kind of funny and kind of sad how all I had wanted was the attention and the compliments, but now I want anything but that. I want to be out of the spotlight now, when before that was all I dreamed about. Now I want to be just another face, blending into the audience. All I want is to not be noticed. To me, being noticed now represents a negative thing."

"Georgia Huston?"

"Yes?" I stood up.

"Dr. Zeltzer is ready to see you," the nurse said. My parents and I followed her.

Mira was already there waiting for us. There was a video camera in the corner capturing the whole room. "Hey guys!" she greeted us.

"Hi Mira," I smiled; I was really starting to like her. "Here's what I have so far." I handed her some of the video tapes that I had recorded.

"Great." She put them in her purse. "Thank you so much."

Dr. Zeltzer walked in. "Hello everyone."

"Hi," we said, sitting down.

"How's everything going?" she asked leaning against the counter.

"Pretty good," I said.

"You've been doing better than pretty good," my dad said smiling.

"Yeah," my mom enthusiastically agreed.

"Okay," I laughed, "I haven't passed out in like a week and when I feel a panic attack coming on I use my hypnotherapy." Mira and Dr. Zeltzer were both taking notes.

"Wow," Dr. Zeltzer said. "That's great! That's just what we want."

"I know. She's doing really well," my dad said proudly. "And tell her what else you're doing," he hinted.

"What do you mean?" I asked, clueless.

"School…" he reminded me.

"Oh yeah!" I remembered, "I've started my courses for school. I take one of the finals tomorrow."

"For which class?" Dr Zeltzer asked.

"World geography."

"Fantastic, and how did that class go?"

"Pretty easy," I said.

"It looks like you're doing great." She seemed pleased.

"I'm doing all right," I smiled proudly. The positive recognition from Dr. Zeltzer gave me even more motivation to keep going.

In total frustration I looked through my closet. I wasn't just trying to find an outfit, I was trying to find an outfit to wear to Notre Dame. I was hoping that no one I knew would be there. That was the reason I'd scheduled the test after school. But if they were there, I was going to look good.

I thought being back on campus would bring a flood of memories but, as I made my way to Mr. Klee's office, I was sad to see that I didn't have flashbacks or anything. I remembered my normal days there, but I wasn't feeling the way I'd expected to feel coming back onto campus. Honestly, I was really feeling like an outcast. I sensed that I no longer belonged there. *Maybe I shouldn't come back here next year after all.*

Everyone in the office was really nice and welcoming to me. I took the test in Mr. Klee's office and he signed everything and mailed it off. I was done with my world geography course; *one down, four more to go.*

When my dad picked me up after the test, Jaron was in the car. He was always popping up and surprising me.

"How'd it go?" my dad asked.

"Pretty good, I don't think I aced it, but I definitely passed," I answered while putting on my seat belt.

"Good, that's all we need – a pass."

We knew I wasn't going to get straight "A's;" I wouldn't have even gotten them if I was still in school. We were just trying to get me to pass the ninth grade so I could get back to school in the fall. In a way that took some of the pressure off, but then again I only had a short time to do everything, so that left plenty of pressure.

My mom hung up the phone when my dad and I walked through the door. Her eyes were red. *Has she been crying?*

"Who was that?" my dad asked.

"Azmi," she said. My dad nodded and left. *What's going on?*

"Are you okay, Mommy?" I gave her a hug.

"Yes, sweetie, I'm fine," she said, forcing a smile and hugging me back. "How'd the test go?"

"It went okay. I'm gonna go lie down for a little. My back's starting to bother me."

"Okay, honey. Do you want me to rub you?"

"No thanks. I think I'm going to try some yoga."

I felt free, after being imprisoned by this pain for so long. I was finally feeling my pain, but not freaking out. Whenever my pain came, I knew how to deal with it. I didn't enjoy having it, but I loved the feeling that I would get after fighting it off and winning.

I really can do this.

After about half an hour my mom and dad went into their bedroom and closed the door. I wanted my mom to play Monopoly with me so I waited for a while, but then I got impatient.

"Nakks, do you want to play Monopoly?" I asked politely.

"No," she said, not even looking up from her book.

"Please, Veronica," I whined.

"No," she snapped.

"Why not?"

"Because you always win and because I don't want to."

"You will get an extra five hundred dollars to start out the game and you can put anything you want on the TV."

She weighed her options for a moment and then slowly put her book down. "Fine."

We went into the living room and played Monopoly together while watching TV. We played for a few hours and then Veronica finally quit; I don't think I ever finished a game of Monopoly with her, but it didn't matter anyway because I was winning by a lot.

I was getting hungry and it was past dinner time so I went looking for my mom. They were still in their room with the door closed. I immediately started assuming the worst because when my parents go into their room for long periods of time, that means something's really wrong. The only times they do that are when someone is in the hospital or when someone dies; the two worst things possible.

I hesitantly knocked on the door. No answer. I knocked again and my dad asked, "What?"

"Is mom in there?"

"Yes, what is it?" he seemed very impatient.

"Can I come in?"

"We'll be there in a second," my mom called through the door.

About ten minutes later my dad came out and went down the hall to my sister's room. When he came out with Veronica, my mom came out of her room. *Everything's okay, nothing happened.* I tried to reassure myself with every positive possibility, no matter how ridiculous, that I could think of.

In the back of my head for some reason I could sense that everything was fine and I knew that I was making a bigger deal of it than I needed to, but I couldn't help it. *What were they talking about in there?*

My parents sat down, so Veronica and I followed suit. Both of them looked exhausted and lost; my mom had been crying again.

"What's going on?" Veronica asked. I couldn't even speak; the tension in the room was scaring the hell out of me.

"We just got some news," my dad said really slowly. I could tell that he was choosing his words very carefully which alarmed me even more. "Your mom got tested last week and it turns out she has a tumor."

"Where?" I asked rudely.

He paused and took a deep breath. "Her heart."

I started crying. "What are you talking about?"

"She has a tumor in her heart, but everything's going to be okay."

"How?" I looked over and noticed that Veronica was crying, too.

"I'm having surgery next week," my mom said, fighting tears.

"Heart surgery?!"

She nodded.

I could feel my face getting red with anger and frustration. "How could you lie to me?!" I screamed at her, "You lied to me!"

"Georgia!" my dad yelled, standing up, "stop it."

"She lied to me!" I pointed at her sobbing.

"What are you talking about?" he asked.

"I asked her why she got tested and she told me nothing was wrong!" I had never felt so betrayed in my life.

"Nothing was wrong." She was pleading for me to calm down.

"Stop lying to me! There obviously was something!"

"Georgia," my dad shouted, "go to your room!"

I gave my parents the dirtiest look that I could and stormed off to my room, slamming the door behind me. I ran onto my bed and jumped onto blankets. I put my face in the pillow and screamed. *This is what Mira wants, right? Emotion?*

I turned on the video camera. I didn't know if Mira would be able to understand me through my tears, but I was going to tape it anyway.

> RECORD:
> "So a couple of days ago I saw a letter from the hospital for my mom and I asked her what it was. She said 'nothing.'"
>
> "Today my parents have the nerve to tell me that she is having open heart surgery next week because she has a tumor," I said with as much resentment as one person could possibly have – then I broke down crying.
>
> "I can't do this Mira, I can't. I'm scared." I whimpered a little, "I can't lose her… I can't be the one to kill her. If something happens it's all my fault because… because I gave her the tumor."

There was a knock at my door. I hit PAUSE.
"Go away!"
I turned back to the camera and lowered my voice.

> RECORD:
> "Isn't that how someone gets a tumor – from extreme stress? I am her extreme stress. I'm killing my mother."

I cried harder that night than I had in a long time.

The next morning I avoided my mom like the plague. She didn't try to talk to me and I didn't talk to her. She seemed really sad and I felt bad for her, but honestly I couldn't get her betrayal out of my mind. It wasn't a little white lie that she told me, like saying my hair looked good when it didn't. This was a big one, a matter of life and death, and I couldn't believe that she would lie to me about something this important.

I'd had a lot of pain that night while I was trying to go to sleep and unfortunately that pain transferred over to the next day as well. Maybe it was because of my stress level or maybe it was going to come anyway, but no matter what the reason was, I just wanted it to end.

There was a knock at my door. I said, "Go away," but the door opened anyway. In walked my dad.

"What do you think you're doing?" he said sharply. I was taken aback.

"What do you mean?" I asked.

"You are being mean to your mother, who just found out she has a tumor in her heart," he said accusingly.

My eyes started to water, "She lied to me."

"Suck it up!" my dad interrupted. "Get over it!"

"But –"

"No," he shook his head, "there are no buts here. Your mother needs you and you need to be there for her. I'm not asking you, I'm telling you."

Then it hit me. *What was I doing?* My dad was right, I was being insane. Part of me wanted to blame it on the drugs that we were still trying to flush out of my body, but the other part was disappointed in myself. I was the one who acted that way and it completely disgusted me. *I'm a horrible person.*

I got up and went into my mom's room where she was lying in bed watching TV. I silently closed the door behind me, crawled onto the bed and grabbed her, crying. We both lay there crying, not saying anything. There was nothing to say, there were so many emotions going through us I wouldn't even know where to start. I was so scared.

The last thing I wanted to do was study, but my dad came in after a couple of hours and told me that I should get back to work. My deadline was going to come up faster than I would think. I knew I should study, but I stayed in there for hours before attempting to do my work. I was going through physical and emotional pain, so I wasn't looking forward to doing anything, but I had to if I wanted to reach my goal and keep my promise. That was the whole thing about chronic pain; I had to keep going, no matter what.

I decided that next I was going to try to get through algebra. I had gotten an 'A' in it the previous semester, but that was with the guidance of an incredible teacher. I didn't know how this was going to go, but I was determined to make it work.

It was surprisingly easy to learn math on paper, because the only thing that I really need is a lot of different examples, which they gave. I did a couple of lessons that day and passed the quizzes. As hard as I tried to focus on my work though, all I could think about was my mom; my sick dying mom; *who I am killing.*

Chapter Thirty-three

"Have you thought of your mantra yet?" Beth asked while I was in the downward facing dog position.

"Sorry?" I had no idea what she was talking about.

"The thing I told you about before, that calms you down and keeps you peaceful," she reminded me.

"Oh my gosh, no I totally forgot. I'll do that today," I promised.

"Okay, do that because it really helps," she said. "How has your pain been?"

"Really bad lately." I started to get a lump in my throat as I tried to explain why. It was so hard to say, "I just found out that my mom has a tumor in her heart."

"No." Beth was utterly shocked. "Is she going to have surgery?"

I nodded, "Next week."

"Oh my gosh," she shook her head in disbelief. "How are you holding up?"

"Not well," my eyes started to water. "I was just starting to get better and now everything's getting worse and there's nothing I can do about it."

"Yes there is," she put her hand on my shoulder. "I want you to start going on walks."

Huh? "Why?"

"Because it will set time aside for just you and you would be getting some exercise also. It's a good way to calm down and reflect. Just do me a favor and try it."

"Can I walk with my dogs?" I had never really been on a walk all alone.

"Maybe in the future, but for right now I would say just go by yourself. Once you get healthier and stronger, we can bring the dogs into the equation," she said. "But seriously, work on a mantra."

When my dad picked me up from Beth's, he handed her some cash. *Doesn't insurance pay for this?*

In the car I asked him, "How much does insurance pay for all this?" He looked at me, then looked back at the road. "None of it."

"What do you mean none of it?" I asked alarmed. "Don't I have health insurance?"

"Yes, you have health insurance, but the insurance company doesn't recognize these therapies as health related. To them they're recreation."

"But isn't my pain real? Aren't I really sick?" I knew what he was going to say, but I thought maybe hearing the answer again would make me start to believe it.

"It is completely real." *Nope, still don't believe it.*

"So we pay for all of this out of our own pocket?" I asked, shocked.

"Unfortunately."

Great, so not only am I killing my mother, but I am running through all of our money, too. Thanks to me we are going to be living on the streets. I hate myself, I truly do. All I do is ruin everything.

When I got home I decided I was going to go on that walk I'd promised Beth. I knew if I didn't do it then, I probably wasn't ever going to. I put on my tennis shoes and put my hair up, I was all set. When I told my dad that I was going on a walk, he asked if I was okay going alone. I said I was, but I secretly wasn't sure if I would be okay. The last time I went on a real walk was when we were out with Jojo and Sean; I ended up passing out mid-step and falling onto the sidewalk. But whatever, I had to face the music sometime. I had to get my life back, and I was willing to face as many bruises as it took.

I started down my street, breathing in the fresh air and soaking in the bright sun; *LA weather is the best.* It had been a while since I'd looked around at my neighborhood. There was a new house being built a block away and the big tree in the front yard of another house wasn't there anymore. That was just another reminder that life goes on, with or without me. *Nobody cares.*

Okay, I've got to make a mantra. I took a deep breath and continued walking down the vacant road. I was surprised at how peaceful it was. *What are the things that I really want in my life? I want to be happy, to experience joy, to be loved, and to have peace. Happy, joy, love, peace... No, that doesn't sound good. Happiness of the spirit... joy of the mind, no joy of the heart, love of the... body and umm... peace of the mind. Happiness of the spirit, joy of the heart, love of the body, and peace of the mind; that sounds pretty good.*

I repeated it to myself a few times and I had a little rhythm going. I was liking this mantra thing.

Where's the fire, what's the hurry about?
You'd better cool it off before you burn it out
You've got so much to do and
Only so many hours in a day

The fire isn't only in my back and leg anymore, it's also in my soul. While the fire in my back and leg are bad, the fire in my soul is good; it's strong. The fire in my soul is the fire in me that is trying to win. It's trying to beat the bad fire. If you fight fire with fire, can one win? Or does it just make a bigger fire? The hurry is that I want to get back to school this fall, I have to. I can't cool it off yet, I have to keep fighting. I won't stop until I have reached my goal and kept all my promises. I might burn out, who knows, but at least I am going to burn out trying. I do have a lot to do in a short amount of time, but I can do it. I can face this challenge and I can win... Can't I, Billy? Can't I have everything?

RECORD:
"Hi, Mira. It's Friday and today I went to yoga and when I came home I went on a walk by myself. That was a big step for me, so I'm actually kind of proud of myself, even if it's really just a tiny accomplishment."

"Beth asked me to make something called a mantra so I made one; don't make fun of it. It's 'happiness of the spirit, joy of the heart, love of the body, and peace of the mind.' The idea behind it is that whenever I get stressed or feel overwhelmed, I say that to myself and then I calm down. I don't know if it'll work, but you know me, I'm desperate for some relief."

"Does anyone else ever feel like they need a break from being them or is that just me? I don't mean to ramble, but when I watch people walking by me I think about how lucky they are. I used to envy their nice clothes and their fancy cars, but now I just envy that they can walk without a limp. I envy their health and how little they have to worry about it. In a way though, I also resent them for it. Is that bad?"

"The thing is that they take it so for granted that sometimes it hurts me. They don't understand what it's like to be dependent on other people to the extent that you need help getting up to go to the bathroom. They don't know what it's like to not be able to take a shower by themselves or what it's like to wake up face down on a sidewalk. They have no idea the hurt and despair that I feel on a regular basis."

"I know I told you that I am going to stop feeling bad for myself, and I really have for the most part. But, I am embarrassed to say that every once in a while it will sneak into the back of my mind. I try to push it out again, but sometimes I do think about it."

"Enough is enough, I'm fine. I will get better, even thinking or talking about it makes me breathe faster and heavier. It stresses me out because I know what I am supposed to be doing and feeling, but it's so hard to feel that way sometimes. Sometimes it's just hard...."

I was rambling and my heart was racing as I started to get more and more frustrated with myself.

I closed my eyes and mumbled, "Happiness of the spirit, joy of the heart, love of the body, and peace of the mind..." over and over again.

"This is a very strong piece of artwork," Esther said, and I was happy because she seemed to be genuinely impressed.

I smiled, "Thank you."

"Have you done a lot of painting?"

"No," I laughed, "I hate painting."

"Wow," she said leaning it up against the wall. "Tell me why you painted this."

I looked at it, one of the boldest pieces of artwork I thought I had ever done. "Well, you have to understand what I'm going through. I recently realized that now that my mom is sick, it's time for me to step up and be there for her the same way that she was there for me. I need to be strong for her like she was for me, and loyal and helpful. I need to be whatever she needs me to be, and I can do that, I think. I can be strong for her even though I'm not very stable. I can fake it." She was listening intently.

"The big hand in the middle of the paper is making a peace sign. All I want is to find peace in all this chaos. If I find peace, I think I will be all right. The red background, yellow lines going through the center, and the purple edges all represent different emotions. They are all bold and distinct colors that, in my opinion, show strength and confidence. I am hoping to find a good balance between peace and strength, so I guess that's what this picture is about."

"Are you the only one you want to find strength in the painting?"

I thought about it, not really understanding the question. "I mean if anyone else can get anything positive out of this, I say go for it, but other than that I don't know."

"Do you think maybe this could be a message to your mother, telling her to continue to be strong?" She was laying her analysis out for me.

"I guess it could be. Maybe it could motivate her," I said, kind of excited.

"I think it would really motivate her," Esther hinted.

"Could I take it home?"

"Can I bring it to the team meeting tomorrow and then give it to you at our next appointment? I think everyone would really enjoy this."

"Yeah, that's fine." I felt a little embarrassed about her showing it to other people, but I didn't really care since they were all part of this process in one way or another.

At my next hypnotherapy appointment, Kathryn mentioned seeing my art. "I was really impressed, I had no idea you were so talented," she praised me.

"Thank you," I smiled.

"We were all so impressed by the way you did the hand. Hands are so hard to draw. I can't even imagine how difficult painting one would be. You have a real gift."

"Thank you."

"Okay," she said enthusiastically, "today I want to try something new. I want to work with energy."

"What does that mean?" I asked.

"Well, you're going to lie down and I'm going to sit right behind you, right in that corner. I am going to take my hands and not touch you, but be as close to your skin as possible, again without touching. The goal is that as I trace up and down your body with my hands, my positive energy will flow into your body as I take your negative energy out. Does that make sense?"

"Yeah," I lied.

I honestly had no idea what she was talking about and thought she was crazy for thinking that she could input her good energy into my being. That was ridiculous.

She turned on some relaxing music, got all set up, and started the "energy transfer." I told myself to stop being skeptical and to be open to the idea that this might work. I fooled myself into believing that this was real, and it actually started to work. I could feel her hands around my body. Even though she wasn't touching me, I knew exactly where she was. It felt as if I really could feel her energy flowing into mine. It was weird. I didn't know if it was just my mind playing tricks on me since I was so desperate, but whether it was all in my head or if it was real, it worked and that was all that mattered.

I finished my algebra course faster than my world geography; I understood math pretty well. I didn't have to worry about scheduling that exam to avoid other students at Notre Dame because it was summer vacation for everyone so they wouldn't be there. *When's my vacation?*

I decided that since I was almost halfway through June that I would try to double up classes. I chose to work on biology and Spanish next – big mistake. I don't know why I chose to do my two worst subjects at the same time, but I did. I was able to fake my way through part of biology. I didn't understand any of it at all, but I did figure out how to memorize it and study for the quiz. When it came to the final for that class, I just winged it, with Mr. Klee over my shoulder. That was nerve racking, but I got through it.

Spanish on the other hand was a complete nightmare. It was impossible to learn a language through a book. I knew nothing and I still don't know how I managed to pass that class. That was the final that I was most worried about and we were waiting on pins and needles for the results, because I was in danger of not passing that class. I ended up getting a "C-" but as my dad kept saying, "All we need is a pass."

Chris came over later and we celebrated; I was over halfway done with my classes. We asked Chris if he could do half an hour massage for me and then the other half for my mom, since she desperately needed the relief. He said of course, but he ended up giving both of us almost forty-five minutes. He was such a nice guy, and an amazing masseuse.

"Can you see if Mira can take you to Esther's tomorrow?" my dad asked.

"No." I hated asking people for any favors. I always thought I was being a bother.

"Georgia, we really need her and she said to call if we had any conflicts. I have to take Veronica somewhere tomorrow and your mom has to go to the doctor. The office is near Esther's, so you can go with your mom if Mira can pick you up when you're done. It's perfect."

I asked, and of course Mira agreed.

I didn't know why my mom was going to this doctor, and honestly I didn't want to know. It's not that I didn't care, I just didn't want to know. I didn't want to hear all the things that were wrong with her, all the things that I caused.

I waited for Mira in the doctor's lobby, and when she came I hopped in her car. She took me to Esther's.

"Explain to me why you picked all these pictures and put them in this way," Esther said, referring to my collage. "I really like it."

"Thanks," I beamed. "You told me to use the magazines to make a collage representing myself. The background images are pieces of fancy jewelry. They make me think of glamour, because I lost all of that to my pain. I felt so unattractive and I hated it, but now it's in the past which is why it's in the background. In the upper left-hand corner there is a big white watch – for time lost on this experience and time that I know I have left to regain the life I want. Next to it is a ladybug for luck, because I could have really used some when I was struggling. There's a bundle of pink flowers because flowers have always made me happy and they are there to remind me to appreciate the little things in life."

"There are also seven people in this collage, all expressing different emotions. One is a woman splashing water on herself – that shows my frustration. There's a girl just staring out into nowhere – that's my confusion. There's a woman sticking her tongue out, showing my silly and fun side – but she's hiding behind the flowers, just like my fun side used to be hiding. At the bottom of the page there are two feet showing relaxation, because everyone loves to relax. There's a soldier of some type in a defensive stance, like he is ready to stand up for himself, even if it means putting up a fight. I'm ready to fight for my health and to reach my goals, so in a way I am a soldier like him. Beneath him is a girl who's laughing and dancing because I love to go crazy like that and just have fun. Then in the left lower corner, there is a woman turning away from the camera, covering her face. That shows the shame and humiliation that I felt, even though I know now that I shouldn't have felt that way. Out of all of those, that was my strongest emotion at the time – shame and humiliation. But, like the soldier, I will stand up for myself and I will fight."

"Do you feel like you have to be all these different people?" she asked.

"I didn't put them there because I feel like I have to be all those people; I feel like I'm already them. I think everyone is like all those people. They are universal emotions that can be used for anyone," I explained. "Someone in China still feels the same emotions as someone in Africa. Wherever you go, a person is a person, a feeling is a feeling."

Esther ended by giving me back the painting of the hand that I wanted to give to my mom.

Just like she'd promised, Mira was waiting outside Esther's door when I came out. "So did your mom call you?" she asked as we boarded the creepy elevator.

"No, she said that she would call when she was done," I said looking down at my phone. "I guess she's not done yet."

"Okay, so what do you want to do?"

"Oh no, I can wait here, or in the lobby of the hospital," I said.

"No, I'm not just leaving you," she laughed.

"But really, I'm fine," I argued.

"But really, I want to stay," she insisted.

She bought me lunch at a little café and we just sat there talking for a while. I will never forget that, because it was the first time I saw them make a cool design with the foam on my hot chocolate. It was so fancy that I didn't want to drink it.

My mom still hadn't called by the time we were done, so – we were in Beverly Hills – what else was there to do but shop? I thought it might be a little awkward, hanging out with a college student I barely knew, but we just kept getting closer and closer every time we hung out.

We walked around and looked at shops. We criticized furniture and we tried on clothes. When my mom called I was actually sorry that we couldn't keep hanging out. I actually felt like a normal teenager for a couple of hours, and I realized how much I missed it and wanted to feel that way again. Being a normal teenager was fun.

Chapter Thirty-four

I went to get a haircut one day that really changed my view of myself. I'd had curly hair my whole life and this new guy asked if he could straighten it. My parents had always been against me straightening my hair, so I only had it done at my friends' houses three times before. I told him that he could do whatever he wanted. I had nothing to lose.

By the time he was done I had side-bangs, something that I never thought I could pull off, and my hair was straight. I didn't recognize myself in the mirror at first, but that was partially what was so appealing about it to me. When I looked in the mirror I saw a different girl, a pretty girl. I had the kind of hair that the girls in the magazines had and that gave me a new sense of confidence.

My parents were not happy with my straight hair at all, but I really didn't care. They begged me to stop straightening it, but I couldn't. I didn't want to go back; I was the new and improved Georgia. I really did feel like a different person when my hair was straight.

I started to wear make-up also. Before that I had just been wearing some mascara, but now I started wearing eyeliner, eye shadow, the whole nine yards. I wasn't wearing sweatpants any more, I was wearing shorts and v-necks. I was determined that if you saw me in a crowd you wouldn't see a sick girl anymore – you would see an attractive girl; someone you wanted to get to know. I thought that by changing my whole appearance I would be leaving my past behind, but there is no way to escape the past.

The past is one of the most important things to a person, because the way you deal with your past determines what your future will be. Covering up a mess in your past just makes a bigger mess, like sweeping everything under the rug. It just makes a lump for you to trip over.

I opened the blinds in my room and started up the camera.

RECORD:

"Hey, so today is a very exciting day," I smiled. "This is my first night back in my own bed in my own room. I haven't passed out in a while, so we all got to move back to our usual sleeping arrangements. I think that's pretty cool. In the living room I was always in the middle of the room so I never really got to look out the windows. This window is staying open all night."

"Living in LA, we don't get to see many stars at night. It seems like every star in the sky is out tonight."

"When I was little I was afraid of the dark, and I'm not gonna lie, but sometimes I still get paranoid alone in the dark like a little kid. I can see how the dark can be scary, but without the dark we can't see the stars. Maybe that's like my life, maybe this experience was for a reason. Maybe I was put in the dark for so long, scared and alone, so that when the stars did show up, they would mean that much more to me."

"It's just an idea… but I can tell you this much – now that the stars are out, I'm never closing this window and going back into the dark again."

The night before my mom's surgery, my sister, mom, and I were in the living room watching movies. We were all there awkwardly trying not to think about the next day.

I had an idea.

"Can I give you guys makeovers?"

They both protested but I finally persuaded them to trust me. I straightened their hair and did their makeup. I took bows and headbands and made their hair in really pretty styles. I took pictures of them and I had fun dressing them up, probably more than they enjoyed getting dressed up, but it took our minds off the next morning.

When I kissed my mom good night, I pretended like it was any other night. I wasn't going to see her in the morning because she would be gone, but I was going to see her that day, right?

Am I going to see my mom again? Of course I am, what am I talking about? I'm just saying good night, I will see her soon. She will be fine… won't she? I kissed her cheek and gave her a little hug. I'll see you soon Mommy.

I looked into Mira's video camera.

RECORD:

"Honestly, I'm more scared about my dad. If you saw him you would think he was the one with the tumor. He's a mess. I wish I could take some of his stress, but I can't. I don't know how he does it, he can't be human. But really, if you saw him and my mom it would seem like he was the one going in tomorrow to have his heart sliced open. I'm worried about him. I'm worried about both of them. There's nothing I can do but wait for my dad to call me tomorrow. It's going to be the longest morning of my life. I can't do anything but wait, and you know how much I love waiting."

I woke up and looked around the house for my parents, just to see if maybe they were there, but they weren't. *6:26: two hours and four minutes until...* I couldn't even say it.

Our family friend, Levie, was doing us a favor and taking me to yoga. I was not in a good mood; all I was doing was watching the clock. I don't know what I was watching it for, there was nothing I could do, but at the same time that was all that I could do – wait.

I had been taking Beth's group classes lately because I was pretty good at yoga now. Beth knew what was going on and I had a feeling some of the other ladies did, too, but I really didn't care. One lady I barely knew came up to me and told me that she was sending my family "white thoughts." I had no idea what that was, but I accepted it. It sounded helpful and we needed all the help in the world.

Levie picked me up after yoga and took me back home, where Pam was waiting for us. I felt bad because I was in such a bad mood to everyone, but I really didn't care. Pam told me to pack because Veronica and I were going to her house for a couple of nights.

Does she know something that she's not telling me? I deserve to know.

My dad finally called. He said that everything was okay, but when I asked if we could go see mom, he said not yet; maybe tonight. *Why can't I see her now?*

Pain shot down my right leg like an angry lightning storm and I fought back tears. I was determined not to cry in front of Jenny.

Pam, Jenny, Becky, and Tom did their best to try and distract Veronica and me, but there wasn't anything they could do. There wasn't anything anyone could do.

It was dark before we finally got the okay to go see mom. I was shaking the whole ride there, trying to imagine what she was going to look like. We were all in our PJs, but no one cared.

Walking through the hospital for someone else was a completely different feeling than going in for myself. I always felt like I had no idea what was going on when I was a patient, but I discovered that when you are just visiting, you know even less. My mom wasn't in her own room, she was in the "intensive care" unit; *that makes me feel better.*

My dad came out to meet us. *If she's okay then shouldn't my dad look better than he does?* He told us that only two people could go in at a time and that we had to lie about Veronica's age so she could see mom. He asked who wanted to go in first. I did.

On the walk down the halls he told me how she might not look that great, but she's doing better and not to worry. That just made me worry more. He asked if I was ready before he pulled back the curtains and I nodded, knowing full well that I was not ready.

He pulled them back, and nope – I wasn't ready. I had been in hospitals before, and I had seen some things. My grandparents used to be in the hospital almost every two weeks, but this was so different that it was staggering. I definitely wasn't ready, but it was too late.

"Hi mommy," I smiled and walked in confidently. I took two steps before my legs started to shake and my stomach started to churn.

"Hi honey," she whispered. It looked like she was trying to smile, and she might have felt like she was, but that wasn't a smile. She always tried so hard to put on a front.

"How are you feeling?" My eyes started to water as I looked down at my frail mother. She had tubes going through her arms, hands, chest, and neck. They were everywhere I looked and each one seemed to have a different color fluid going through it. Her eyes could barely open and there was gunk all over her mouth. Only half her consciousness was there in the room with me.

"Great," she said sarcastically.

I felt the tears running down my cheek; *suck it up! Be strong for her.* "Is there anything you need?"

"Yeah," she said slowly and took a deep breath. She was speaking really slowly. "Can you wet a towel with some cold water and put it on my forehead?" She wasn't making a whole lot of sense, but I understood.

I went over to the faucet and while I was wetting a towel I wiped my tears away; *be strong.* I put it on her forehead like she asked, but all I could look at were the tubes in her neck. I had never seen that before. She attempted to make a little smile again and she grabbed for my hand. I almost threw up when she held my hand because that wasn't her hand. That wasn't my mom's hand. *My mom's hand doesn't have tubes in it.*

I really started to lose it.

"I'll go send Veronica in, mom," I smiled through my tears. I was certain that even with her eyes closed she could tell that I was crying through my voice. "I love you, mommy. Have a great night." I looked for a spot to hug her, but there wasn't one. I kissed her forehead and opened the curtain to go out. "I love you Mommy."

"Bye, sweetheart."

I got out in the hallway and literally collapsed. I fell to the floor like I had just gotten the wind knocked out of me. My dad came after me and Pam came running, too. Jenny stood up and Veronica turned into Becky's arms, sobbing. Pam grabbed me and picked me up. She held me as I cried and moaned. I wasn't worried about being loud, I didn't care that the security guard was looking at me weirdly. I had never cried so hard or loudly in my life as I did after seeing my mom for the first time.

My back was killing me; *of course I would get pain right now. Go away fake pain. Fuck you fake pain.* "I can't do this," I stuttered into Pam's shoulder, "I c-can't do this."

"Shh…" she said rubbing my back. "Yes you can, she's fine. Your mom's fine, honey."

"No, no, no. You didn't see h-her. She's n-n-not-t fine."

"Everything's okay," she said.

"No, nothing's ever okay."

I sobbed to the camera.

RECORD:
"I can't do this, Mira. It's just hit after hit for me. Any time things start to go well, something happens like this."

"What I'm mostly upset about is that I wasn't there for her. But, I couldn't be. I'm an awful daughter; I couldn't spend more than ten minutes with her. I should've sucked it up. I hate myself. She spent all night with me when I was in the hospital and I couldn't even be bothered for ten minutes. But it was just so sad to see her like that."

"I guess that's how everyone felt when they saw me in bad shape. This just makes me push even more; I don't want to make other people feel the way I feel when they look at me. I don't wish this feeling on anyone. I need to keep my promise. No more hospital beds for me."

The next day was the Fourth of July; *joyous occasion, right?* Pam, Jenny, Becky, and Tom took Veronica and me to a park to watch the fireworks. There was a big fair going on with different stands of food and games. A band played on the stage and it was very crowded.

I saw a guy I knew from Notre Dame when I walked in, and skillfully dodged his line of vision. I laughed at myself because even if he'd seen me, there was no way he would have recognized me. That's what this whole make-up and hair straightening thing was about; a new, unrecognizable identity.

Jenny and I walked around and socialized. It was really fun, and I felt normal. I felt really guilty that I was out having a good time while my mom was stuck in a hospital bed, but that's the way she wanted it. She wanted us to go tonight.

While we were lying on the grass and watching the fireworks, I thought about my mom and how maybe somewhere out there she was watching the same fireworks I was; maybe.

When Jenny and I went back to her house, we stayed up all night talking to guys on the phone and video-chatting. I couldn't help but blush as they told me how pretty I was. Every guy I talked to that night asked for my number, which just further encouraged the hair straightening and makeup. I was finally getting positive attention from boys; *me, the awkward girl in the body cast.* I went to bed with the biggest smile on my face. Things were changing.

My dad called in the morning and told me that they had moved mom into her own room.

"I thought last night was supposed to be her last night?" That got me worried.

"It was. Everything's fine, though," he said. "They just want to keep her for observation." In adult language that meant that something was wrong.

"Wow, the flowers are really pretty," I said as we all crammed into my mom's new room. "Who are they from?"

"Mely, bless her heart," my mom smiled. "She stopped by this morning." Mely was our nanny from the time I was two until about fourth grade, and we have stayed friends with her family.

"That's nice," I said. "I made you something, too." I handed her the painting of the fist that I made with Esther, but my mom couldn't really hold it so I put it on the window sill. She was still having a hard time moving around.

"That's really pretty, honey. Is it for me?"

"Yes," I laughed.

"Oh, thank you, Peaches," she said holding her arms out for a hug. I gave her a hug and for some reason it wasn't so hard this time.

"I also," I started searching through my bag, "brought you some pictures." I pulled out a bunch of frames.

"Are those from our living room?" mom asked as I put them up around her room.

"Yes," I smiled.

"Thank you, honey. That's very sweet. You guys just missed Briana," she said and pointed to a box on the table. "She gave me this necklace."

I opened the box and saw a silver chain with a heart on it. In the heart was a tree, the tree of life. It was a really cool design and I loved the way it was styled. "That's so pretty."

"Yeah, but I can't wear it while I'm in the hospital."

"I'll take care of it for you," I said, gently putting it around my neck.

"Well okay then," she laughed. "Will I ever get that back or is it going to be like when you borrow my clothes?"

"It's some incentive for you to get better. You'll get to wear this when you are out of here. I promise."

I yawned into the camera for my daily video diary.

> RECORD:
> "Hey Mira. Today I saw my mom. She's better I guess, but she was supposed to be released yesterday. Instead they admitted her, so I don't know what's going on. I can tell there is something they're not telling me, but no surprise there. She is still really weak, but she seems to be more alert…"
>
> "There's something new going on in my life… I've started to talk to boys again – well actually they're talk-

ing to me. I'm texting three of them at the moment. I don't really know what has changed, but I like it. It's so different, I'm really not used to it. I'm getting a lot more confident now, maybe I am pretty. Maybe I won't be the girl with the limp anymore, but the girl who makes heads turn. Just a thought. I know that won't happen, but it's nice to dream... I'm happy, Mira. I am really genuinely happy."

I put my headphones in my iPhone. Now I could listen to music whenever I wanted. I smiled as I turned up "Vienna" and continued to text my new friends.

Slow down, you're doing fine
You can't be everything you want to be
Before your time
Although it's so romantic on the borderline tonight
Tonight....

I'm slow, I'm relaxed, I'm happy. I can finally say that yes, I am doing fine. But the thing is, Billy, that it <u>is</u> my time. It's now my time and I can be everything I want to be. Romance can mean a lot of things, but who knows... maybe I will start up a few romances of my own. Not tonight, but soon; hopefully very soon.

Chapter Thirty-five

Mira picked me up in the morning and dropped me off at Beth's. When I was done getting my yoga on, we had almost four hours to kill so Mira decided she was going to take me out. We went to the mall together and had lunch at the food court. We talked and laughed and I showed her pictures of all the boys I'd been talking to. She said they were very cute and asked me what they were like. I gossiped about them and told her who played what sport or went to what school. She laughed and told me how she missed her high school days.

I told her that I did, too.

After lunch we went downstairs and I got a milkshake; I was in the splurging mood. *Who wouldn't be with a life like mine?* It was an outdoor mall in Brentwood and was absolutely enormous. We walked around and I asked her if she wanted to try on some dresses. We went into store after store, picking out as many dresses as we could carry, and dragged them into the dressing rooms. We would try them on and then model them for each other. I would tell Mira how much I loved her style and she would tell me what a great figure I had. She was honestly becoming such a good friend and it was weird because I was never really reminded of the age difference. She really treated me with respect and like an equal.

Then Mira took me to Kathryn's. Kathryn noticed at once how much happier and more positive I was. As I drifted off into the abyss, I had to fight a smile. Things were finally going my way.

The next day Jenny and I went shopping. We went around the mall trying on clothes just like I had with Mira. I was surprised at how differently we were treated while trying on the clothes than Mira and I were treated. People change so much according to who they are with. When salesmen see an adult, they see a sale; in kids all they see is extra clothes they'll have to put away later. While that is usually true, for some reason it bothered me. *Why do Jenny and I deserve less respect than Mira and*

I? Kids deserve respect, too.

When an adult interacts with an adult, their body language is naturally more respectful and dignified than when they talk with a child. A child is lesser in their eyes, not in an impolite way, but in a matter of fact way, and therefore they hold themselves differently. Just like when sales clerks see a child they think "burden," when doctors see a child they might think "whiner." *Why do adults judge children just by their age?*

Kids aren't taken seriously, which was one of the big problems that I went through. If an adult went to a doctor and said they had pain, I think the chances of the doctor looking at them and telling them they are making it up to get attention is much less than if a child said it; or a teen... maybe a teen like me.

Before I fell asleep that night I was lying in my bed looking up at the ceiling. Naturally my eyes soon shifted over to my ceiling fan. I laughed because I had always been so embarrassed by that fan, but loved it at the same time. When someone entered my room they wouldn't see my bright green bed sheets or my walls covered with the stunning Joe Jonas and the smoking hot Ryan Gosling first. No, their attention would go straight to my ceiling fan.

We moved to this house when I was in sixth grade, and the first week we were living there my fan broke. The landlord said he would take care of it, and knowing how much I loved baseball, got me a fan that he thought I would love. I came home from school to a baseball themed ceiling fan, literally.

The light globe was a giant baseball and the base of the fan was a huge glove holding the baseball. The actual fan blades were four blue, yellow, and gray bats spinning around. Where the fan mounted into the ceiling was a home plate. My jaw dropped.

Needless to say, the fan didn't exactly fit in with the whole teenage girl vibe I had going on in my room, and I got teased about it by everyone, but in a way I loved that fan. Every time I looked at it I had to laugh, but in a way it worked. It showed who I really was.

Looking up at the baseball light in the glove, with the bats spinning around home plate, I thought back to my baseball career. I thought about my grandpa and how much he wanted to watch me play softball for Notre Dame. Such a simple request, and I was determined to get on the team. I was going to make him proud.

"Hi Mommy," I said coming into her hospital room.

"Hi honey," she smiled and slowly tried to sit up, but remained lying down.

"How are you feeling?" I asked.

"I'm doing okay. How was the fourth of July?"

"It was really fun. Did you get to watch fireworks?"

"No," she said looking out the window, "I didn't see any. I could just hear them."

"Aw, well I took plenty of pictures," I started flipping through the pictures from that night on my iPhone.

"You took pictures of the fireworks?" my dad asked, laughing in the corner.

"Yes," I gave him a look. "I didn't know if mom would be seeing any so I took pictures for her just in case."

"That's so sweet," my mom smiled looking at all my pictures. "Thank you, baby."

"Hey Ms. Georgia," Jojo said smiling when I met her in front of my house. "You ready?"

"Yes ma'am," I smiled. That weekend was Phyllis's birthday and Jojo was throwing her a surprise party. It was going to be a costume party, the theme being the decades of her life. We were going to go shopping at some of the vintage clothing shops near my house and find costumes for the party. We didn't end up finding anything that we wanted, but it was really fun looking around with her and trying on funky old clothes.

I knew I had to get back to my school work. I only had two more classes to do, so I started my English course. The quizzes were on some reading that I was issued and there was a big essay that I had to turn in at the end as a major part of my grade. It was the longest time I'd spent on one single class because it was really boring and I didn't want to work on it. *There has to be more to life than these courses. There is more to this world than grades.*

When I got out of yoga, Jojo and Sean were waiting patiently for me. I was feeling good after such a difficult class, it felt so good moving around and working my muscles.

"Hey guys," I said cheerfully when I got in the car.

"Why hello there, Ms. Georgia," Jojo said smiling.

"Hey Sean," I said turning back to him, but he was hiding behind the cape he was wearing. "Is Sean not here?" I asked playfully as Jojo drove.

Jojo played along, "I thought I brought him, I guess I didn't. That's too bad because I thought we could all go out to breakfast."

"To where?" I asked.

She looked at me and smiled, "IHOP?"

"You know me too well," I laughed.

"I want to go to IHOP!" Sean burst out from behind his cape.

Jojo and I both pretended to be startled. "How long have you been back there?!"

After breakfast we went to the grocery store to get some things for Phyllis's surprise party. While we were there we got my mom an orchid because she loves them.

When we got back to their house we played with clay and drew pictures. Sean is really creative and artistic so we were a perfect match. That evening I went to a concert at the Hollywood Bowl with Sean, Jojo, Russ, Phyllis, and Henri. It was really fun and it felt great to get out and do stuff. I slept over at their house.

It came out of nowhere.

"Kristy's softball team needs another player for a game tomorrow," my dad mentioned casually. "Jerry asked if you could fill in."

"Is Jerry the coach?" I asked.

"No, he's not. It's a club team, though."

"I really don't want to," I said.

"I think you should. Just go out and give it a try. What do you have to lose?" he pressed.

"Do I have a choice?"

"I think you should go," he hinted.

"Fine, but I haven't played in over a year."

"They know."

I hung out with Kristy the next day. We stayed at her house for a little bit and then walked around Ventura Boulevard. It was really fun, but the whole day I was thinking about the game that I was expected to play in. I was so nervous that I was going to show up and suck. I wouldn't be able to handle that.

When I arrived I was almost shaking. Kristy blended right in with all her friends; *but would I?* The girls were really nice to me and I did the warm-ups just fine. I played catch with Kristy and I was surprisingly accurate. I was impressed with how little my throw had changed.

During the game I wasn't a star, but I was a star in my own eyes for a change. I didn't stand out compared to the other players, but I did so much better than I'd expected. I didn't strike out; I got on base every time. Every ball that was hit to me, I played perfectly. I played really well, but to me – I played amazingly. I was so happy with how I was doing. I couldn't help but smile when I was at second base; *I'm back.*

They asked me to join the team so I guess I did pretty well. I told them I'd get back to them. I had never really played competitive softball before. I'd been on teams and in tournaments but not an intense club team like this. I didn't know if I was ready, but if they offered me a spot I guess I was.

"Hello?"
"Hey grandpa," I said happily.
"Hello?"
"Hi, it's Georgia," I said a little more loudly.
"Oh," I could hear him smile, "Georgia."
"How are you?"
"I'm good."
"How's grandma?" I asked.
"Oh, she's good. I had them do her hair and nails today." He always wanted her looking her best and got mad at the nurses if they didn't do her hair the way he wanted it.
"That's sweet."
"Yeah, yeah. It looks pretty good," he said.
"So guess what I did today."
"What?"
"Played softball."
I could feel his mood lighten. "Really?"
"Yeah, I played for a club team. They asked me to join," I bragged.
"Really?" he sounded so excited. "Is it for Notre Dame?"
"No, it's for a different team."
"So you're not going to play for Notre Dame anymore?"
"I'm going to try," I explained. "Their team starts playing in the spring, so until then I might play for this one."
"That sounds good," he replied sounding happy.
"I just wanted to call and let you know that I'm back," I grinned.
"Back at what?" he asked.
"I'm back at softball, I'm going to be back at school. I'll be back at everything."

"Can't wait."

"Tell grandma I say 'hi,'" I said.

"Okay dear, love you."

"Love you, too, Grandpa."

I completed my English requirements and passed the final exam. The last course that I had to do was my elective, which was a PowerPoint class. I had always understood how to use PowerPoint, so we thought that I could get through it pretty quickly.

"Can we do that energy thing again?" I asked Kathryn as I sat back in my chair.

She shrugged, "If that's what you want."

She came and sat over me. I took deep breaths, each one sinking deeper and deeper into nowhere land. When I drifted away, for some reason the first color I'd always seen was black, but this time I saw white. I'd never noticed that I always saw black first until it wasn't there anymore. It was just something I'd accepted and never really questioned. *Can I control what color I see or is this just a coincidence?* Maybe that was a metaphor for how I was feeling. Maybe I was in the dark before, but now I see the light; now I can see.

I felt Kathryn's positive energy flowing through my body and mixing with mine. I felt our happiness and joy blend together and make something special. I felt elated; I could finally see the light.

Chapter Thirty-six

I put on my purple v-neck and my navy shorts. Jenny finished straightening her hair while I did my make-up. For some reason I was a little nervous; I didn't know why since it wasn't a date.

When we got to the movies we all got our popcorn and drinks. We talked and laughed in our seats while we waited for the movie to start; "Transformers 2." Jenny and I had never seen the first movie, but David and Harry had – that's right, we were with boys.

While we were watching the movie I couldn't help but smile. It wasn't a date, I didn't have a crush on either of them, but I felt like a teenager. I was beginning to feel that way a lot lately and I liked the feeling.

I only had a couple of weeks left until school started. I sat down to finish my PowerPoint course, following all the guidelines and clicking on all the right buttons. It was really long and tedious, but it was actually pretty easy. I was walked through all the steps; it was a joke, but after all the hard courses that I'd struggled in, I wasn't about to complain.

I went to visit my mom in the hospital one day and when the nurse came in I went out into the hall. I overheard what was really going on. My mom's heart's rhythm was not normal, so that's why she wasn't able to leave the hospital yet. If it didn't fix itself by the end of the week they were going to have to restart it with an electric shock. My palms got sweaty when I heard this. *I thought the surgery went fine, what else aren't they telling me?*

I always seemed to leave yoga feeling proud of myself. Beth was always pushing me to do things that I never thought I could do, but it turned out that I could. I was going through that a lot lately also. I was starting to realize that I could do more than I thought I could. I was surprising myself with how much better my life was getting.

Dawn and Sarah picked me up and I slowly got into the car; I was so sore, but again, it was a good sore. We went back to their house and hung out for a bit. We played with the ball and with dolls. Sarah loved playing doctor so she would bring out her doctor kit and pretend to perform surgery on me. Sometimes she would actually put the toy thermometer in my mouth or pretend to cut into me a little harder than she should have, but I always played along.

At one point she pretended to give me a shot and I pretended to be unconscious. I closed my eyes and lay down on the floor. She didn't move for a moment, I could feel her watching me. *She's not being a very good doctor.* After a couple of seconds she got up silently and ran into the other room. I got up and followed her, trying not to laugh.

"Sarah," I said, "I'm right here. Where are you going?"

She was relieved. "I thought you went to sleep again, like before."

My heart dropped. "Don't worry Sare Sare, I don't go to sleep like that anymore."

My dad picked me up from their house that evening. While we were driving back in rush hour traffic I thought about Sarah and how sensitive she was now whenever I closed my eyes. *Did I ruin her childhood? Is she going to think that everyone playing pretend with their eyes closed has passed out and that she needs to get help? Did I change her?*

"Dad! Dad!" I ran around the house looking for him.

"What?" He came running in. "What is it?"

I jumped into his arms and hugged him, "I'm done!"

"Done with what?" he asked.

"School!" My eyes started to water, "Call Notre Dame." I took a deep breath and whispered, "I'm done."

I was feeling goofy, so Jenny and I went out to Studio City. We walked around the shops and decided we wanted to have some fun. We picked out the ugliest clothes we could find. We put articles together that no one would have even imagined. We tried to hide our laughter as the people working at the stores gave us strange looks while we put on polka-dot skirts, zebra tops, and knitted scarves. We even ended up buying this huge ugly flowered skirt that was three dollars. It was the largest skirt we had ever seen; both of us tried it on together when we got to my house. We looked in my mirror, taking pictures and laughing at how silly we looked. While looking in the mirror I noticed the "7/11" in the corner and felt proud. I was keeping my promise. I was going to reach my goal, I was sure of it.

We cut the ugly skirt in half, still big enough to wear if we stitched it back together, and took out Sharpie markers. We wrote our favorite quotes on it and all our inside jokes. We drew pictures and had fun designing it. I felt some pain in my leg, but I was able to fight it off using hypnotherapy without Jenny even knowing. I was getting pretty good at that. The best part was that I wasn't just pretending like I wasn't feeling the pain, I was able to manipulate it so that I really couldn't feel it.

Now I could tell the camera my deepest, darkest feelings.

> RECORD:
> "I control my pain, Mira, no one else. People can tell me to do stuff and how to react, but it doesn't do any good unless I decide to do it for myself. It's like when a drug addict's family and friends are begging them to quit, but they aren't going to quit for good until they decide for themselves that they want to stop using. If the family tries to cut them off, they will most likely just find other ways to get it. The only way to beat an addiction is to genuinely want it to be over. My addiction was feeling sorry for myself; it's an easy thing to do. So, the challenge is dealing with it and getting better. It was a challenge, and I don't want to jinx it, but I don't know, Mira, I think I might be getting better. I just might be getting back to normal."

"Georgia," my dad said brightly, "your mom's coming home tomorrow." He was smiling.

I smiled back. "That's great."

"So, this house needs to be clean by tomorrow morning. It's up to you and Veronica to get it done."

Ugh. Veronica and I spent the day cleaning. We made the house look as nice as possible and even decorated mom's room a little because we knew she was going to be spending most of her time in there. *Mom is almost home.*

"Does that mean her heart's beating normally now?" I asked my dad.

He gave me a look like I wasn't supposed to know that, but I could also tell that he really didn't care that I knew. "Yeah, they restarted it today and it's back to normal. Everything's fine."

I sighed with relief. "Good."

"You got the okay from Notre Dame today. They have approved all your course requirements and you're going back when school starts at the end of the month," he said giving me a pat on the back.

"Really?" My face lit up.

"Wasn't easy was it?" he laughed.

"Not at all."

"But you did it."

"I guess I did."

"How are you doing?" Esther asked when we sat down.

"I'm doing great," I said glowing. "My mom comes home today."

"Really? That's great, she smiled, and I heard you're going back to school, too. That's so exciting. We're all so proud of you."

"Thanks, I'm really happy."

"So do you remember, one of your first appointments with me, I had you draw a self-portrait?"

"Yeah," I only vaguely remembered it, "I guess."

"Well, I want you to draw me another one," she requested.

"No mirror?" I asked laughing.

She nodded, "No mirror."

When I was done using the pastels I leaned my latest self-portrait up against the wall like always. For some reason I felt kind of embarrassed. It didn't look like me.

"This is your self-portrait?" Esther asked surprised.

I nodded.

"Why do you illustrate yourself in this way?"

I cringed when I looked at it. I was looking at myself as an old lady. "I feel like this whole thing has aged me desperately. I feel a lot wiser, but at the same time I feel like I've lost my innocence. I grew up since the beginning of the year. I've grown up more than I was supposed to over a year. I didn't age with wrinkles or gray hair like the self-portrait. I aged emotionally. I lost years that I can never get back, but like I said before, I'm wiser because of it. I matured, for better or for worse, and now that I've accepted that I can move on."

I looked back at the future me on the paper. The only thing that anyone could associate with me was the bright blue eyes. *Maybe I'll look like that one day.*

Slow down, you crazy child
and take the phone off the hook and disappear for awhile.
It's all right, you can afford to lose a day or two
When will you realize... Vienna waits for you?

Slow down, smell the flowers. Nothing is so important that I should go crazy over it. I can take the phone off the hook because I come first. I should always come first. When I need a break, I need to take it. I can't put too much pressure on myself or all my progress will just be backtracked. I know, Billy, I know; Vienna's waiting for me. I'm close to getting there, just hold on a little longer; please, I'm almost there.

When I heard the gate open and close my heart nearly jumped out of my chest. I ran to hug my mom, but she put her hands up to stop me. "Honey, I'm sorry but I'm kind of fragile right now." *Was I not allowed to hug her?*

My mom sluggishly made her way into the house and then into her bed. Watching her move so slowly was painful because my poor mom was suffering She was going through so much and it was killing me.

Mira came over to give my mom a little stuffed heart. My mom had a collection going of heart related objects.

She hadn't taken a proper shower since before her surgery so she asked if I could help her.

I said, "of course."

That was the first time I saw her scars. She had some holes in her stomach area where the tubes went in and I could see the area where they split open her ribs. I'd never done well with blood or cuts so I just tried my best not to look without being rude.

When I was standing over her, washing her matted hair, I thought about how the roles used to be reversed. She had been the one taking care of me and taking showers with me. Now that she needed help, I was there for her; just like she'd been there for me.

Chapter Thirty-seven

As I walked into the lobby and rode up the elevator of the all too familiar building on the UCLA campus, I thought back to my prior visits. I thought back to the time I'd limped up the driveway on my crutches, and the time that I passed out walking out of the elevator and my dad caught me. I remembered seeing those halls for the first time and the crowded waiting room. It was all so strange to me then, but now it was my comfort zone. This was the place that saved my life.

"Hi Mira," I said hugging her. She was already waiting in the room with her video camera set up.

"Hey guys, how's Lynn?" she asked.

"She's doing better," my dad said sitting down.

"Thank you so much for the heart. That was so sweet," I smiled.

When Dr. Zeltzer came in I was overwhelmed with a strange feeling. I was feeling extreme gratitude. I wasn't just looking at some doctor. I was looking at the woman who not only single-handedly gave me my life back, but also taught me how to keep it. Dr. Zeltzer and her team listened to me when no one else was. They didn't give me another number and tell me to take a seat, they asked me how I was feeling and gave me my identity back.

"Hi guys, I'm so happy to hear that you're going back to school soon," Dr. Zeltzer said.

"In three days," I gloated.

"That's so exciting," Dr. Zeltzer smiled. "Are you still taking your Lexapro?"

"Yeah, shouldn't I be?"

"Yes, we'll keep you on that for a little longer," she said writing something in her notebook. "How's your mom?"

"She's great, thanks."

"Do you have any questions for me?"

"No, I really don't."

"Well, do you think you are on the right path?"

I laughed, "I think I am directly on the right path."

"And you're even starting to play softball again," she smiled back. "That's great."

"Thanks." It felt good to be praised by someone like Dr. Zeltzer.

"I have a question for you, but don't feel like you have to say 'yes.' UCLA is doing a study for kids with chronic pain. They are calling it the Peer Mentor Study and the idea behind it is to help kids going through this feel less alone. If you were to agree, you would go to a training session as a mentor, and then you'd be assigned a mentee. I don't know the details exactly, but you'd talk on the phone with kids about your experiences. You help them through their treatment. If you're interested I can put you in contact with them."

"That would be amazing. I would love to do that," I said, overjoyed.

She smiled. "Really?"

"Yeah," I said. "I really, really want to."

"Great, I will let them know," she looked at me admiringly. "Gosh, I just cannot believe you. Look at you, Georgia. You are such an incredible woman. You are going so many great places."

"All thanks to you," I said.

She shook her head, "No, it was all you. We just showed you how to do it."

"I cannot tell you how much you guys saved me."

"It was our pleasure, really. Everyone loves you."

"Well thanks," I blushed.

She looked at me and laughed. "You should write a book about all this."

"No one would read that." I laughed, too.

"You'd be surprised."

At the end of that appointment, when we said 'goodbye' and when I watched her leave the room I couldn't help but get choked up. I knew that wouldn't be the last time I saw her, but I couldn't help but get emotional. I thought back to all those doctors who told me I was crazy and the other doctors who wouldn't even give me the time of day. I thought about how with the help of Beth, Esther, Kathryn, Chris, and Dr. Zeltzer, I'd found my way back. Every doctor or professional that I saw, I would beg. I would pray that they would be my hero. I would say to myself, *Doctor, be my hero.*

I found my heroes.

"Can I borrow your glasses?" my mom asked, in a sexy black dress and heels. She was all done up, hair and makeup.

"Okay," I said pointing at her, "What'd you do with my mom who came home from the hospital yesterday?"

She laughed, "Who?"

"Of course you can use my glasses, Mrs. Jackie O," I said handing her my big sunglasses.

"Why thank you, Ms. Hippie," she joked back.

It was the night of Phyllis's surprise costume party. My mom had just gotten home and she was already going out to party; she was amazing. When we got to the party no one could believe that she'd just had open heart surgery. She looked so good and she was so lively. She had a few moments of discomfort, but for the most part she hid it well.

She didn't sit in bed and feel sorry for herself; she got up and carried on with her life. She did exactly what I'd had to do, but she figured it out a lot faster than I did. I was so proud of her for getting better. *See, nothing to be afraid of. My mom can take anything.*

"Guess where I'm going tomorrow," I said to my grandpa.

"Where?" he asked.

"School," I said proudly. "Notre Dame High School."

His face lit up. "How?"

"I finished my ninth grade year and I'm going back."

"Good for you, Georgia," he smiled. "That reminds me," he said standing up and going over to his bedside table, "I have a newspaper article for you about this girl who goes around teaching boys how to play baseball. Boys are actually paying her to teach them," he laughed.

"That's very cool," I smiled, "thanks Grandpa." In the stack he handed me there were also a couple of silly comics; *of course.*

Chapter Thirty-eight

As I zipped up my high waisted khaki skirt I closed my eyes and remembered when I couldn't even zip it over my body cast. I put on my white polo with the "ND" on the left and thought about how lost I was when I lost that community. I put on my tall white socks and tied my tennis shoes, hoping that I could find my way around the campus. I put on my "NDHS Knights" sweatshirt that I got the first night I attended a Notre Dame event. I looked in the mirror and saw my straight hair and long eyelashes. *Will anyone recognize me?* I hoped they wouldn't, but I knew it was just a matter of time.

I knew I would be asked questions about everything under the sun, but I also knew that it would be completely worth it. I knew that Notre Dame was where I belonged and the second that I walked on that campus, I felt like I was home. I was glowing when I walked to my locker. I was back at school and normal. I made it. I kept my promise.

"Oh my God! Georgia is that you?!"

I walked up the stairs and into the room with the long table and chairs. I was the first one there so I sat down and waited patiently. One by one they came in and took their seats. We awkwardly smiled at each other. After a couple of minutes some adults came into the room.

"Hello everyone and welcome to the Peer Mentor Study Training."

It was more therapy for me than it was training. That day I met six other teenagers, five girls and one boy, who were all within a couple of years of my age. We were all athletic, creative, smart, and social people; we all had chronic pain.

We sat around that table exchanging stories and feelings about what we went through. We had never met before, never even knew the others existed until that day, and all had almost identical experiences. We spent seven hours in that room, relating to complete strangers. None of us could believe how similar all the things we went through were. We were all alike. We were all united.

We all talked about how alone we felt and how much it would have helped if we had known each other during our struggles; if we'd known anyone who went through what we did. It was such an inspiration for me to meet them and I will never forget that day.

Steve and Talia picked me up after the training because I was sleeping at their house that night. I got in the car from the pouring rain, put on my seat belt, and I broke down.

I wasn't crying out of sadness or out of pain. I was crying because I was so relieved. I cannot describe the way I was feeling with words, it was too overwhelming. I watched the water droplets race down the window, paralleling the tears racing down my cheeks.

I'm not crazy.

Meeting those six people has changed my life forever. They showed me that there were other people out there like me, and they need help, too. Even though my pain was under control at that time, I finally realized what chronic pain was and what it meant to me. For the first time in over a year I realized that I was not alone; I never was.

> *You've got your passion, you've got your pride*
> *but don't you know that only fools are satisfied?*
> *Dream on, but don't imagine they'll all come true*
> *When will you realize, Vienna waits for you?*

I found my passion, Billy; I found what I am supposed to do. I was meant to go through all this, there was a reason for it. My passion is to help other kids going through chronic pain.

I have so much pride, which I never thought I would be saying. I am proud of myself and I am happy with who I am. I am strong and I am a fighter. You're right, only fools are satisfied. I am not a fool.

I am not going back to the way things were, I'm going to make things better. I never used to dream, but now that I can dream again, I'm never going back. I can't ignore my dreams anymore because they are here for a reason.

Kids with chronic pain won't be alone anymore. Why can't all my dreams come true? Who's going to stop me? I have been waiting for Vienna for as long as it has been waiting for me. I finally realized, enough waiting; I have to find it.

And guess what, I did. Vienna is not a place that I can drive or fly to; it was in me the whole time. Vienna is different for everyone. For some people it could be a vacation to Hawaii or snowboarding down a mountain in Colorado. For me, it wasn't a destination or activity. After two years of searching, I finally found my Vienna.

I have happiness in my spirit, joy in my heart, love for my body, and peace of my mind.

I have my life back.

Vienna can stop waiting; I'm ready now....

Acknowledgements

Dad – You never doubted me. You fought for me when no one else would. You believed in me even when I didn't. You will never know how much you mean to me. I can say it over and over again, I can tell the world, but no one will ever fully understand.

Mom – You lay with me for hours, holding me, crying. You let me break down in your arms, you let me feel. You were there in a way that no one else was; I just always knew that you were on my side. Your sacrifices did not and do not go unnoticed. Your constant strength inspires me. I can only dream of being as strong as you one day.

Nakka – For all the times I yelled at you when you didn't deserve it – for all the times you waited at school or missed soccer practice – for all the things I put you through; I'm sorry. I'm sorry you had to go through what you did; I wish I could give you back that year. My childhood wasn't the only one that ended; I wasn't the only one who was forced to grow up. You are the unsung hero of my story. I'm sorry for everything.

Dr. Lonnie Zeltzer – You are the voice for those who can't be heard; the hope for people that can't see it. Your incredible faith in others motivates everything I do. You gave me my life back, along with so many others. You are one of the most generous people I know; generous with your time and with your love. You were never just a number; you are my doctor. My family and I owe everything to you. Never stop what you're doing.

Apateece, Dawn, Talia, and Sarah – We are meant to share everything with our family; the good times and the bad. You have unfortunately seen both. You have seen me at my best, but you have also seen me at my worst. Through everything you have loved and supported me just the same. Thank you for always being there for me.

Jojo, Russ, Phyllis, Henri, and Sean – You really stepped up. You have always been in my life and always will be. You are my family. I will forever be grateful for all you did and continue to do for me. You will always have a special place in my heart.

Tom, Pam, Jenny, Becky, and Janice – You always knew how to get my mind off things. You didn't feel bad for me; you had me get up and do stuff. You made me forget, even if it was just for a little while.

Beth, Kathryn, Esther, and Chris – My angels. I trusted you with my deepest emotions and secrets and you never let me down. I turned to you in my darkest times and you always gave me another way to deal with it; a better way to look at things. There is always another way. Thank you for showing me that.

Zane – No one understands me like you do; no one believes in me the way you do. When I break down you always find a way of picking up the pieces. You push me even when I fight you on it. You tell me how great I am when I don't want to hear it. You make me a better person. You keep me going.

Andy and Terri – You have always been my biggest art fans and have stimulated my creative side for as long as I can remember. Even when I was a toddler drawing with markers, you always saw potential and didn't treat me like a little kid drawing stick figures. You made me feel like an artist, so that's who I became. My art success is due to you; you are the ones who make me want to continue art.

John and Carla – You have continued to support my family and me through everything. I wish you could only know how dear you are to me and how much I value our friendship. Thank you for everything.

Grandma and Grandpa – Your love was not shown through hugs and kisses, it was shown through your actions. You always stood up for your morals and taught me to stand up for mine. I think of you all the time; every day. You showed me what true love and dedication are. Your commitment to each other encourages me. Grandma, I wear your ring every day and will never forget what it stands for. Grandpa, I played for the Notre Dame softball team; we did it. I wish you could have been there to see all my accomplishments but you are always with me. With every comic clip I find and every hummingbird that flies by, you are with me. You are desperately missed but lovingly remembered. I hope you found your Vienna; I hope you are at peace.

About Georgia Huston Weston, LCSW

A longtime sufferer of chronic pain, Georgia wrote this book while a student at Notre Dame High School. She also founded the Teen Pain Help Foundation, a 501(c)3 charitable corporation created to help children and adolescents with chronic pain. Georgia then served as the Executive Director, raising funds for treatment, research, education, and increased public awareness of pediatric chronic pain.

Afterward, she attended St. Edward's University in Austin, Texas, where she received a Bachelor of Arts in psychology, with a minor in art. As a student she worked as an intern counseling at-risk children and youths for the state of Texas, and she helped seniors and the mentally challenged with art projects. She also wrote a second book on pain.

Georgia went on to receive a Master of Social Work degree from the University of Southern California, with a concentration in Children, Youth, and Families, as well as a focus in Child and Adolescent Mental Health. She also co-founded and was the Director of Programming for Art Rx, strengthening the partnership between the USC Suzanne Dworak-Peck School of Social Work and the USC Keck School of Medicine, specifically to better understand how art impacts pain.

Georgia has experience creating and leading programs for organizations that provide therapeutic services for struggling individuals and families. She also has clinical social work experience, both as an outpatient therapist and residential therapist, for youth dealing with complex cognitive, behavioral, and social needs. And, she has been a Research Associate with the UCLA Pediatric Pain Research Program.

From 2019 through 2022, Georgia served as the Executive Director of Creative Healing for Youth in Pain (CHYP), a nonprofit that provides educational resources, creative healing experiences, and social support for youth with chronic pain and their parents (*www.mychyp.org*).

In recognition of her humanitarian services, Georgia received the David Chow Humanitarian Foundation Award for 2019.

A Licensed Clinical Social Worker, Georgia currently works as a mental health therapist. And, she is the author of two other books on chronic pain.

Also by Georgia Huston:

The Smart Brain Pain Syndrome

Co-authored with Dr. Lonnie K. Zeltzer and Dr. Paul M. Zeltzer, *The Smart Brain Pain Syndrome* (2021) provides a new approach to chronic pain in children and young adults. Longtime pain sufferers are guided through a clear and unexpected explanation of how pain can come from the brain. The solutions are not typical medical prescriptions and therapies, but instead are a wide variety of creative outlets that soothe and retrain the brain, providing relief.

PAIN: An Owner's Manual

If you hurt, read this book!

A young pain victim's inspirational and informative conversations with a variety of pain sufferers and specialists. They share their experiences with pain, their coping strategies, and what works for them in getting through the day.

Astonishingly frank conversations range from marijuana use to music therapy to suicide. A must-read for all doctors, who will get an earful from the other side of the examination room. They offer honest revelations about living with pain caused by Fibromyalgia, Chronic Regional Pain Syndrome, Irritable Bowel Syndrome, Arthritis, Postural Orthostatic Tachycardia Syndrome, Migraines, Ankylosing Spondylitis, Thoracic Outlet Syndrome, Arnold Chiari Malformation, Cerebral Palsy, and more.

Different therapies and coping strategies work for different people, ranging from video games to noise canceling headphones to working out, watching TV, Botox injections, or performing standup comedy. For some, it's creating art, for others it's riding horses, or petting their dog.

There are realistic discussions of therapies such as biofeedback, Iyengar yoga, and hypnotherapy. And candid revelations about drugs -- from pot to brand name prescription narcotics -- and tales of addictions, young and old. Horror stories turn into hopeful tales of personal heroism, perseverance, family unity, and caring.

Doctors should read this at their own risk.

Printed in the USA
CPSIA information can be obtained
at www.ICGtesting.com
JSHW051551260224
57591JS00010B/63